CAH Screening

CAH Screening—Challenges and Opportunities

Editors

Natasha Heather
Anna Nordenström

MDPI • Basel • Beijing • Wuhan • Barcelona • Belgrade • Manchester • Tokyo • Cluj • Tianjin

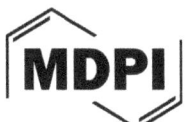

Editors
Natasha Heather
University of Auckland
New Zealand

Anna Nordenström
Karolinska University Hospital
Sweden

Editorial Office
MDPI
St. Alban-Anlage 66
4052 Basel, Switzerland

This is a reprint of articles from the Special Issue published online in the open access journal *Actuators* (ISSN 2076-0825) (available at: https://www.mdpi.com/journal/IJNS/special_issues/cah).

For citation purposes, cite each article independently as indicated on the article page online and as indicated below:

LastName, A.A.; LastName, B.B.; LastName, C.C. Article Title. *Journal Name* **Year**, *Volume Number*, Page Range.

ISBN 978-3-0365-0924-2 (Hbk)
ISBN 978-3-0365-0925-9 (PDF)

© 2021 by the authors. Articles in this book are Open Access and distributed under the Creative Commons Attribution (CC BY) license, which allows users to download, copy and build upon published articles, as long as the author and publisher are properly credited, which ensures maximum dissemination and a wider impact of our publications.

The book as a whole is distributed by MDPI under the terms and conditions of the Creative Commons license CC BY-NC-ND.

Contents

About the Editors vii

Natasha L. Heather and Anna Nordenstrom
Newborn Screening for CAH—Challenges and Opportunities
Reprinted from: *Int. J. Neonatal Screen.* **2021**, 7, 11, doi:10.3390/ijns7010011 1

Aashima Dabas, Meenakshi Bothra and Seema Kapoor
CAH Newborn Screening in India: Challenges and Opportunities
Reprinted from: *Int. J. Neonatal Screen.* **2020**, 6, 70, doi:10.3390/ijns6030070 5

Svetlana Lajic, Leif Karlsson, Rolf H. Zetterström, Henrik Falhammar and Anna Nordenström
The Success of a Screening Program Is Largely Dependent on Close Collaboration between the Laboratory and the Clinical Follow-Up of the Patients
Reprinted from: *Int. J. Neonatal Screen.* **2020**, 6, 68, doi:10.3390/ijns6030068 15

Patrice K. Held, Ian M. Bird and Natasha L. Heather
Newborn Screening for Congenital Adrenal Hyperplasia: Review of Factors Affecting Screening Accuracy
Reprinted from: *Int. J. Neonatal Screen.* **2020**, 6, 67, doi:10.3390/ijns6030067 25

Kate Armstrong, Alain Benedict Yap, Sioksoan Chan-Cua, Maria E. Craig, Catherine Cole, Vu Chi Dung, Joseph Hansen, Mohsina Ibrahim, Hassana Nadeem, Aman Pulungan, Jamal Raza, Agustini Utari and Paul Ward
We All Have a Role to Play: Redressing Inequities for Children Living with CAH and Other Chronic Health Conditions of Childhood in Resource-Poor Settings
Reprinted from: *Int. J. Neonatal Screen.* **2020**, 6, 76, doi:10.3390/ijns6040076 43

Rolf H. Zetterström, Leif Karlsson, Henrik Falhammar, Svetlana Lajic and Anna Nordenström
Update on the Swedish Newborn Screening for Congenital Adrenal Hyperplasia Due to 21-Hydroxylase Deficiency
Reprinted from: *Int. J. Neonatal Screen.* **2020**, 6, 71, doi:10.3390/ijns6030071 75

Sari Edelman, Hiral Desai, Trey Pigg, Careema Yusuf and Jelili Ojodu
Landscape of Congenital Adrenal Hyperplasia Newborn Screening in the United States
Reprinted from: *Int. J. Neonatal Screen.* **2020**, 6, 64, doi:10.3390/ijns6030064 83

Phyllis W. Speiser, Reeti Chawla, Ming Chen, Alicia Diaz-Thomas, Courtney Finlayson, Meilan M. Rutter, David E. Sandberg, Kim Shimy, Rashida Talib, Jane Cerise, Eric Vilain, Emmanuèle C. Délot and on behalf of the Disorders/Differences of Sex Development-Translational Research Network (DSD-TRN)
Newborn Screening Protocols and Positive Predictive Value for Congenital Adrenal Hyperplasia Vary across the United States
Reprinted from: *Int. J. Neonatal Screen.* **2020**, 6, 37, doi:10.3390/ijns6020037 101

Mark R. de Hora, Natasha L. Heather, Tejal Patel, Lauren G. Bresnahan, Dianne Webster and Paul L. Hofman
Measurement of 17-Hydroxyprogesterone by LCMSMS Improves Newborn Screening for CAH Due to 21-Hydroxylase Deficiency in New Zealand
Reprinted from: *Int. J. Neonatal Screen.* **2020**, 6, 6, doi:10.3390/ijns6010006 111

Fei Lai, Shubha Srinivasan and Veronica Wiley
Evaluation of a Two-Tier Screening Pathway for Congenital Adrenal Hyperplasia in the New South Wales Newborn Screening Programme
Reprinted from: *Int. J. Neonatal Screen.* **2020**, *6*, 63, doi:10.3390/ijns6030063 . . . . **125**

About the Editors

Natasha Heather is a pediatric endocrinologist based in Auckland, New Zealand, and has dual roles within both newborn screening and clinical endocrinology. She is actively involved with the Clinical Laboratory Standards Institute (CLSI) as chair of NBS11, an upcoming international guideline on newborn screening for CAH. She also chairs the Australasian Paediatric Endocrine Group (APEG) NBS subcommittee, promoting regional co-operation and harmonization efforts. She was the 2018 recipient of the International Society of Neonatal Screening (ISNS) Jean Dussault Medal. Her main research interests are in newborn screening outcome and quality evaluations.

Anna Nordenström is a pediatric endocrinologist at the Karolinska University Hospital in Stockholm, Sweden. She is responsible for the national neonatal screening for CAH. Her research at the Karolinska Institutet is focused on CAH and disorders of sex development. She has conducted studies on neonatal screening, growth, pre and postnatal treatment, fertility, psychological aspects, cognition, brain MRI studies and national registry and epidemiological registry studies on the long term outcomes in CAH correlating the results to the severity of disease using the CYP21A2 genotype. She is actively involved in the I-CAH/I-DSD registries and is active in the European reference network for rare endocrine disorders, RareEndoERN, as a work package lead for quality of care and patient view.

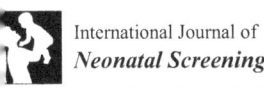

Editorial

Newborn Screening for CAH—Challenges and Opportunities

Natasha L. Heather [1,2,*] and Anna Nordenstrom [3,4,5]

1. National Newborn Metabolic Screening programme, Specialist Chemical Pathology, LabPlus, Auckland City Hospital, Auckland 1023, New Zealand
2. Clinical Research Unit, Liggins Institute, University of Auckland, Auckland 1010, New Zealand
3. Centre for Inherited Metabolic Diseases, Karolinska University Hospital, SE-171 76 Stockholm, Sweden; anna.nordenstrom@ki.se
4. Department of Women's and Children's Health, Karolinska Institutet, SE-171 76 Stockholm, Sweden
5. Pediatric Endocrinology Unit, Astrid Lindgren´s Children's Hospital, Karolinska University Hospital, SE-171 76 Stockholm, Sweden
* Correspondence: NHeather@adhb.govt.nz

Newborn screening for congenital adrenal hyperplasia (CAH) using 17-hydroxyprogesterone (17-OHP) as an indicator of disease was first introduced in the 1970s [1]. Prior to this, the female preponderance among clinically detected patients and the cellular architecture of the adrenal glands had led to difficulty in understanding both the inheritance and pathogenesis of CAH. Following the introduction of screening, it became clear the CAH is a monogenic autosomal recessively inherited disorder with a wide spectrum of phenotypic severity. The female preponderance was explained by neonatal mortality due to early salt crises or hypoglycemia, mainly amongst boys without obvious signs of the disease at birth. Conversely, as affected females undergo prenatal genital virilisation, they are often, but not always, detected clinically soon after birth.

Newborn screening for CAH detects babies affected by deficiency in the adrenal enzyme 21-hydroxylase, which is the most common cause of CAH (>90%). The molecular genetics of *CYP21A2* and the genotype–phenotype correlation of pathogenic variants have been important tools both in studies of the disease and in setting up relevant and effective screening programs. Most screening programs today aim to prevent neonatal salt crisis and mortality. Hence, they are targeted to detect babies with the classic forms of CAH, mainly the salt-losing form. Newborn screening for CAH provides clear benefit in preventing neonatal salt crisis and mortality, especially amongst boys. However, despite substantial benefits and a high uptake of CAH screening worldwide, there are still a number of ongoing issues to be resolved, including:

- Timing of the specimen collection. This is important in CAH, as the result has to be communicated early enough to be effective in preventing salt crisis, yet later samples can detect more affected individuals, albeit with less severe forms of the disease.
- The relatively high false positive rate and a low positive predictive value (PPV) of CAH screening. This is largely due to variation in 17-OHP levels in the neonatal period and in severely ill infants. In particular, immunoassay measurements of 17-OHP amongst preterm infants can be falsely elevated as a result of cross-reactivity with metabolites found in the immature adrenal gland.
- Clinical follow up and the availability of treatment. This is crucial to a successful screening program. Despite hydrocortisone being an inexpensive medication, it is not readily available in all parts of the world.

These issues are not straightforward and continue to be obstacles both to the uptake of CAH new-born screening and to quality improvement in established programs. They require balanced solutions that reflect local healthcare systems and priorities and may, therefore, be resolved in different ways around the world.

On the initiative of the *International Journal of Newborn Screening* (IJNS), the opportunity arose to realise this project, a Special Issue on "CAH Newborn Screening—Challenges and Opportunities". The aim of this Special Issue was to describe the current state of CAH screening around the world, with a focus on efforts to find solutions to obstacles and on successful strategies to improve the efficiency of screening.

We would like to take this opportunity to thank the authors for their excellent contributions and the *IJNS* for their support. We feel the resulting series of articles provides an evaluation of the current status of new-born screening for CAH, and insight into the path for quality improvement across the globe.

Dabas and colleagues [2] report on the challenges and opportunities for CAH NBS in India. India's high annual birth rate results in over 4 million new-borns each year. To date, the only Indian state to provide comprehensive new-born screening is Kerala, a state in Southern India, which commenced screening for CH, CAH, G6PD and galactosaemia in 2012. The incidence and prevalence of CAH in India is not known, although screening pilot studies have reported a variably high incidence of 1:2300 to 1:10,000. Limitations revealed by Indian pilot studies of CAH NBS include high false positive rates, incomplete follow-up of babies with positive screens and limited availability of confirmatory testing and follow-up care. In addition, limited access to maternity care and medical review of new-born babies mean that birth weight or gestational age related cut-off levels, which can generally reduce the false positive rate, cannot easily be applied. The authors describe cultural reasons to conceal gender ambiguity and case series, suggesting high mortality and morbidity amongst those presenting with adrenal crises in infancy, such that the early detection and treatment of affected babies would be expected to greatly improve survival.

The national Swedish neonatal screening programme began screening for CAH in 1986 and has made significant contributions to the global understanding of CAH. In a further review, Lajic and colleagues [3] report that long-term outcomes for patients with CAH can be improved by close collaboration between the screening laboratory and the clinical side. This is because good outcomes from new-born screening do not just relate to early detection and are highly dependent on clinical follow up. The authors demonstrate how the screening laboratory can contribute to awareness of CAH amongst clinicians, to knowledge and information about the disease, and to initial treatment of screen-detected babies with CAH. This collaboration is important in ensuring prompt and sufficient early treatment, as well as to avoid overtreatment. Furthermore, the Swedish National CAH Registry contains data on over 700 individuals with CAH and provides valuable information to support screening evaluation through notification of missed cases or delayed diagnoses, as well as through assessment of long-term outcomes. Long-term results regarding mortality, cardiovascular outcome, cognition and possibly fertility may similarly be improved.

Held and colleagues [4] provide a review of the impact of foetal and neonatal physiology on new-born screening for CAH. Current first-tier screening methodologies lack specificity, leading to a large number of false positive cases, and adequate sensitivity to detect all cases of classic 21OHD that would benefit from treatment. First-tier screening based on immunoassay assessment of blood 17-OHP levels in new-borns lacks specificity, especially amongst preterm babies, leading to a high rate of false positive screen results. Sensitivity may also be inadequate to detect all cases that would benefit from early detection and treatment. The pathology of CAH due to 21-hydroxylase deficiency, the development of the foetal hypothalamic-pituitary-adrenal axis development and adrenal steroidogenesis are all described. The authors highlight five factors that contribute to both false positive and false negative results, reviewed alongside current best practice for specimen collection in the United States and worldwide.

Specific problems that arise for children with CAH in resource poor countries are outlined in the publication by Armstrong et al [5]. Since 2004, Caring and Living as Neighbours (CLAN), an Australian non-governmental organization working to improve the lives for children with chronic health conditions in resource poor countries, has collaborated with a broad range of partners across the Asia–Pacific region in order to improve the quality of life of children with CAH. The treatment of CAH is complex in that steroid doses must be adjusted during infections with a fever and may require hospital care for intravenous treatment in severe situations. Common issues for children in resource-poor countries include access to medication, education regarding medical management, and access to family support groups. This study shows that improvements in quality of life for children with CAH can be achieved using CLAN's approach.

An update of Swedish neonatal screening [6] illustrates the genotype–phenotype correlation in CAH and how that can be used to improve the screening and understanding of CAH. The detection of virtually all patients with the salt losing form and all of those with the null genotype demonstrate the effectiveness of new-born screening. The Swedish paper also illustrates that samples collected later, especially amongst preschool children, facilitate the detection of less severe forms of the disease. Offering screening to children up to the age of 8 years when moving into Sweden led to the identification of a surprisingly high number of children with non-classic and simple virilising forms. These children are obviously not the target of the new-born screen, and the paper raises a valid question regarding whether such children should then be treated with replacement doses of hydrocortisone.

New-born screening for CAH is now performed in all states in the USA, with specimen collection occurring relatively early, and most often between 24–48 h after birth. Furthermore, the Secretary's Advisory Committee on Heritable Disorders in Newborns and Children (ACHDNC) recommends a target of notifying presumptive positive screening results for CAH and other time-critical conditions by five days of life [7]. The Special Issue includes an analysis of screening performance, particularly timeliness, across the USA, based on voluntary data submitted to the Newborn Screening Technical assistance and Evaluation Program (NewSTEPS) data repository [8]. Their report includes > 850 aggregate case counts of CAH and nearly 500 with individual case level data, submitted from 35 contributing state screening laboratories. A key strength of the NewSTEPS data is the use of public health surveillance case definitions to facilitate the consistent categorisation of new-borns. Of note, the median age at release of out-of-range CAH screening results was just 4 days, reflecting considerable success in initiatives to extend laboratory operating hours and facilitate the rapid reporting of out-of-range results.

Within the USA, screening protocols have been adapted and implemented separately by individual state laboratories over the past several decades. The Special Issue includes an overview of 17 of the screening protocols currently used in the USA, illustrating the presence of large differences in approach, as well as screening sensitivity and specificity [9]. Despite using birth-weight-related cut-off levels, reported PPV varied from less than 1 to 50%, and CAH prevalence from 1/10,000 to nearly 1/30,000. Although there was considerable variation in 17-OHP cut-off levels, this did not correlate to either PPV or prevalence. Most state screening laboratories recommend a second sample for infants in intensive care. In addition, there are four two-screen programmes which require a second sample to be collected at two weeks of life, regardless of the result of the first sample, and PPVs were highest amongst these. The authors recommend that quality improvement be directed at the standardisation of protocols across state laboratories, as well as towards enhanced communication between clinicians and screening laboratories, with the eventual aim of achieving a uniform set of best practices.

Within this Special Issue, two Australasian screening programmes report their experience in implementing a second-tier liquid chromatography tandem mass spectrometry (LC-MS/MS) method. De Hora and colleagues from New Zealand [10] report on the performance of a LC-MS/MS method to measure 17-OHP alone. Screening performance was assessed by comparing national screening metrics 2 years before and after LC-MS/MS implementation, within a screened population of approximately 60,000 each year. In the 2 years after LC-MS/MS implementation, the authors demonstrated a four-fold reduction in the overall number of false positive screening tests and concomitant increase in PPV from nearly 2 to 11%, with no loss of sensitivity observed. Furthermore, they noted that the

LC-MS/MS method could be turned around and reported quickly after an initial elevated primary immunoassay test, with results available within 2 h when required.

New South Wales was the first Australian state to commence NBS for CAH in 2018 also using a two-tier protocol. The results of the first 203,000 screened babies are reported here [11]. Samples above the 17OHP threshold level on first-tier immunoassay were further tested using LC-MS/MS, and those with a ratio of (17OHP + androstenedione)/cortisol > 2 and/or 17OHP > 200 nmol/L on LC-MS/MS were referred to as presumptive positive screens. The incidence of CAH detected through NBS was 1:22,551, with a PPV of >70% and no known false negatives. All affected newborns were notified and reviewed clinically prior to the development of an adrenal crisis. In contrast to high false positive rates still reported through screening protocols that rely solely on 17OHP immunoassay levels, this report demonstrates that screening specificity can be dramatically improved through the use of a steroid profile.

We want to thank all the authors for the contributions to this Special Issue, and the expert reviewers for their valuable comments and questions, which were important to the overall quality of the series. New-born screening for CAH has been shown to be effective in detecting infants at risk of developing adrenal salt crisis and thereby decreasing neonatal mortality. It is possible that the screening per se also improves the long-term outcome for these patients in several ways, including increasing knowledge of the disease and its treatment. The authors have provided a state-of-the-art series to help achieve these goals across the globe. Whilst much has been achieved in the field of NBS for CAH, there is clearly still work to do in optimising both the screening approach and outcomes.

Funding: This manuscript received no external funding.

Conflicts of Interest: The authors declare no conflict of interest.

References

1. Pang, S.; Hotchkiss, J.; Drash, A.L.; Levine, L.S.; New, M.I. Microfilter Paper Method for 17α-Hydroxyprogesterone Radioimmunoassay: Its Application for Rapid Screening for Congenital Adrenal Hyperplasia. *J. Clin. Endocrinol. Metab.* **1977**, *45*, 1003–1008. [CrossRef] [PubMed]
2. Dabas, A.; Bothra, M.; Kapoor, S. CAH Newborn Screening in India: Challenges and Opportunities. *Int. J. Neonatal Screen.* **2020**, *6*, 70. [CrossRef] [PubMed]
3. Lajic, S.; Karlsson, L.; Zetterström, R.H.; Falhammar, H.; Nordenström, A. The Success of a Screening Program Is Largely Dependent on Close Collaboration between the Laboratory and the Clinical Follow-Up of the Patients. *Int. J. Neonatal Screen.* **2020**, *6*, 68. [CrossRef] [PubMed]
4. Held, P.K.; Bird, I.M.; Heather, N.L. Newborn Screening for Congenital Adrenal Hyperplasia: Review of Factors Affecting Screening Accuracy. *Int. J. Neonatal Screen.* **2020**, *6*, 67. [CrossRef] [PubMed]
5. Armstrong, K.; Yap, A.B.; Chan-Cua, S.; Craig, M.E.; Cole, C.; Dung, V.C.; Hansen, J.; Ibrahim, M.; Nadeem, H.; Pulungan, A.; et al. We All Have a Role to Play: Redressing Inequities for Children Living with CAH and Other Chronic Health Conditions of Childhood in Resource-Poor Settings. *Int. J. Neonatal Screen.* **2020**, *6*, 76. [CrossRef] [PubMed]
6. Zetterström, R.H.; Karlsson, L.; Falhammar, H.; Lajic, S.; Nordenström, A. Update on the Swedish Newborn Screening for Congenital Adrenal Hyperplasia Due to 21-Hydroxylase Deficiency. *Int. J. Neonatal Screen.* **2020**, *6*, 71. [CrossRef] [PubMed]
7. Secretary's Advisory Committee on Heritable Disorders in Newborns and Children. Newborn Screening Timeliness Goal 2017. Available online: https://www.hrsa.gov/advisory-committees/heritable-disorders/newborn-screening-timeliness.html (accessed on 5 February 2021).
8. Edelman, S.; Desai, H.; Pigg, T.; Yusuf, C.; Ojodu, J. Landscape of Congenital Adrenal Hyperplasia Newborn Screening in the United States. *Int. J. Neonatal Screen.* **2020**, *6*, 64. [CrossRef] [PubMed]
9. Speiser, P.W.; Chawla, R.; Chen, M.; Diaz-Thomas, A.; Finlayson, C.; Rutter, M.M.; Sandberg, D.E.; Shimy, K.; Talib, R.; Cerise, J.; et al. Newborn Screening Protocols and Positive Predictive Value for Congenital Adrenal Hyperplasia Vary across the United States. *Int. J. Neonatal Screen.* **2020**, *6*, 37. [CrossRef] [PubMed]
10. De Hora, M.R.; Heather, N.L.; Patel, T.; Bresnahan, L.G.; Webster, D.; Hofman, P.L. Measurement of 17-Hydroxyprogesterone by LCMSMS Improves Newborn Screening for CAH Due to 21-Hydroxylase Deficiency in New Zealand. *Int. J. Neonatal Screen.* **2020**, *6*, 6. [CrossRef] [PubMed]
11. Lai, F.; Srinivasan, S.; Wiley, V. Evaluation of a Two-Tier Screening Pathway for Congenital Adrenal Hyperplasia in the New South Wales Newborn Screening Programme. *Int. J. Neonatal Screen.* **2020**, *6*, 63. [CrossRef] [PubMed]

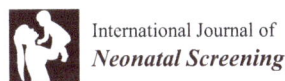

International Journal of
Neonatal Screening

Review

CAH Newborn Screening in India: Challenges and Opportunities

Aashima Dabas, Meenakshi Bothra and Seema Kapoor *

Department of Pediatrics, Maulana Azad Medical College and Lok Nayak Hospital, New Delhi 110002, India; dr.aashimagupta@gmail.com (A.D.); meenakshibothra@gmail.com (M.B.)
* Correspondence: drseemakapoor@gmail.com

Received: 6 July 2020; Accepted: 25 August 2020; Published: 27 August 2020

Abstract: Congenital adrenal hyperplasia (CAH) is a common treatable disorder which is associated with life-threatening adrenal crisis, sexual ambiguity, and/or abnormal growth if undiagnosed. Newborn screening is a cost-effective tool to detect affected babies early after birth to optimize their treatment and follow-up. Newborn screening however is in its nascent stage in India where it is not yet introduced universally for all babies. The following review briefly highlights the challenges (e.g., lack of universal screening, healthcare resources) and opportunities (e.g., reduction in morbidity and early correct gender assignment in females) associated with newborn screening for CAH in a large Indian birth cohort.

Keywords: newborn screening; congenital adrenal hyperplasia; CAH

1. Introduction

Congenital adrenal hyperplasia (CAH) refers to a group of autosomal recessive disorders caused by inherited defects in steroid biosynthesis. It is most commonly caused by a deficiency of the enzyme 21 alpha hydroxylase, leading to the deficiency of mineralocorticoids and glucocorticoids and excess of sex steroids. The disease presentation may be classical, as salt-wasting (SW) or simple virilizing (SV), and non-classical. Classical CAH is most readily discernible when it presents with virilization in girls, but it may be missed in boys, who may manifest with life-threatening adrenal crisis within the first few weeks of life [1].

Newborn Screening (NBS) for CAH

In 2002, the Joint Lawson Wilkins Pediatric Endocrine Society/European Society for Pediatric Endocrinology Working Group recommended biochemical screening for classical CAH in the newborn period to reduce associated morbidity and mortality [2]. Newborn screening (NBS) for CAH is performed by measuring 17-hydroxyprogesterone (17OHP). This is traditionally measured by radioimmunoassay, enzyme-linked immunosorbent assay or time-resolved fluoroimmunoassay. In an effort to reduce the high false positive rate associated with immunoassay screening for CAH, the 2018 Endocrine Society Clinical Practice Guidelines recommend a second-tier screen by liquid chromatography tandem mass spectrometry (LC/MS-MS) [3].

The levels of 17OHP are influenced by maturity, stress, maternal steroid administration and age. Cord blood is easier and non-invasive, but is not recommended for CAH screening as the steroid surge at birth results in significantly higher 17OHP levels which can be difficult to interpret [4,5]. Capillary blood samples (usually collected later by heel prick onto collection paper) are ideal for measurement of 17OHP for NBS. They also provide an opportunity to screen for other disorders of metabolism in the same sample [5,6]. In a study on newborn screening of 3080 babies from Southern India, prematurity significantly increased the mean 17OHP values from 4.86 ± 2.47 to 8.97 ± 7.43 ng/mL and the median 17OHP value from 4.5 to 6.3 ng/mL (measured on competitive immunoassay) [7]. Investigators from different regions of the World have found that sex, mode of delivery as well as seasonality affect 17OHP values [8,9]. Another study from India comparing the 17OHP levels (radioimmunoassay) in sick vs. healthy neonates demonstrated that gestational age, birth weight, and Apgar score were negatively correlated, whereas stress factor, mode of delivery and use of antenatal steroids in mothers were positively correlated with 17OHP levels [10].

India's high annual birth rate of 17.8 births per 1000 results in the birth of over 4 million newborns per year, of which over 277 thousand are home births. Screening such a large cohort would not only need a robust newborn screening program, but also some mechanism to ensure that the babies born at their homes are not missed [11]. In medical facilities with high turnover, babies are usually discharged within 24–48 h of delivery, thereby increasing the chances of inadvertently missing these babies if screened 48 h after birth. The sample collection time for newborn screening for CAH is, therefore, a balance between practical considerations about coverage, the best time to assess 17OHP level and the need to have results early enough to minimize the risk of salt-wasting adrenal crisis. Therefore, we suggest the sample for NBS to be taken at least 24 h later, but may be taken up to day 7 of life, using heel-prick [5]. Preterm babies should be screened at 2 weeks and 4 weeks of age or at discharge from NICU, to decrease the risk of missing a case of CAH [3]. In addition, there should be close monitoring of electrolyte imbalance, blood glucose and blood pressure of babies in NICU.

There may be high false positive rates with the first-tier immunoassay due to cross-reactivity and physiological changes in the concentration of 17OHP during the first few days of life, especially in preterm neonates [12]. Screening specificity can be improved with second-tier testing; for example, LC/MS-MS of steroids including 17-hydroxyprogesterone, 21-deoxycortisol, androstenedione, and cortisol [13]. At present, a LC/MS-MS facility is not available for most screening programs in India. However, it is planned to assign a centralized laboratory for confirming screen positive samples in different districts. Infants positive for the newborn screen test should be referred to a pediatric endocrinologist for evaluation. A confirmatory diagnosis may be performed by cosyntropin stimulation test. Molecular testing is an available option for confirmatory diagnosis in screen positive individuals. It will also help in offering prenatal diagnosis in the subsequent pregnancies. However, cost constraints and limited availability remain major hurdles to its current use in the Indian context.

2. Disease Burden in India and Need of NBS

The overall disease burden of CAH in India is not known but is likely to be significant. CAH remains the most common cause of female ambiguity and primary adrenal failure in Indian series underscoring the magnitude of the problem [14–16]. Most affected newborns succumb to adrenal crisis in their first few weeks of life or early infancy in the absence of a confirmed clinical diagnosis [17,18]. In an Indian report by Rajendran et al., 8 out of 22 (36.4%) unscreened babies who presented with features of salt-wasting CAH in the neonatal period died during infancy, at a median age of 3 months (0.2–13 months) [19]. In a study by Miati et al., there were just 10 males out of a total of 45 children with classical CAH seen at a tertiary clinic, of which, 2 males were noted to have sustained cognitive impairment as a result of multiple episodes of severe hyponatraemic encephalopathy prior to diagnosis. The skewed sex ratio suggests that the affected males with SW-CAH may have died undetected, and that the burden of disease in India is even greater than reported [20]. Virilized female infants with SV-CAH and affected children of both sexes with precocious puberty may not be brought to medical attention for the fear of social stigma, resulting in delayed diagnosis [21].

The incidence and prevalence of CAH in India is not known. However, CAH qualifies for screening in India, as per the Wilson and Jungner criteria as it is seen frequently in our country, is treatable when diagnosed early and might result in irreversible sequelae if left untreated [22]. However, newborn screening is still not being routinely done in India. It has been done intermittently, in project mode, in various studies. Table 1 shows the details of newborns detected to have CAH on newborn screening by various investigators from India. In a multicentric study of the 104,066 newborns screened for CAH, 18 infants (16 SW, 2 SV) were confirmed to have CAH, suggesting a collective incidence of 1 in 5762. The study showed marked regional differences, with the prevalence being 1 in 2036 in Chennai, 1 in 7608 in Delhi and 1 in 9983 in Mumbai [23]. Other recent studies from India, found the incidence of CAH to be 1 in 2800 in South India [24] and 1:6334 in North India [4]. The differences in incidence of CAH reported from India may be because of the variations in technique used, different cut-offs, different disorder definition and/or different populations screened. The incidence figures reported from India are higher than those reported from European countries [25]. This could be due to the high consanguineous marriage rate (1–30%), especially in certain population groups, resulting in higher incidences of recessively inherited diseases. Population stratification into different castes and endogamous mating could also be a contributor [26].

With the Prenatal Diagnostic Act in place in India, identification of gender in the prenatal period is not permitted. The birth of a baby with sexual ambiguity comes with a considerable social stigma for the family. Unless the family is able to conceal genital ambiguity, affected babies are at risk of being whisked away and illegally adopted by Hijra (transgender groups). In India, gender reassignment from 'male' to a 'female' may be difficult for the affected families for fear of stigmatization [27]. The process of registering a change of gender of the baby in the birth certificate can be complex and tiring for the families within the legal framework. Moreover, where female feticide poses an additional danger to the survival of a girl, the change of gender from 'male' to 'female' may not be welcomed in many Indian families, even in the 21st century. The clinicians should therefore assist the parents to assign the biological gender as the gender of rearing in those presenting with ambiguity, as also recommended by most consensus groups [28]. Newborn screening informs early and accurate assignment of biological gender and is of high societal importance in India.

Among an Indian cohort of 81 children (32 boys, 49 girls) with congenital adrenal hyperplasia due to 21 hydroxylase deficiency, two-thirds (57) had salt-wasting and the remaining had simple virilizing type. Twenty-five (31%) of these children had short stature and 45 (55.6%) had growth velocity below the reference range [29]. CAH is not a target disorder for NBS in Great Britain. A two-year nationwide CAH surveillance study in Great Britain reported 144 cases of childhood CAH, of which 86 (59.7%) presented in infancy (37 simple virilization, 30 salt-wasting, 12 affected siblings, 8 others). Fifty-eight subjects presented later at median age of 5.9 years with precocious puberty in the majority (66%) and genital virilization and affected sibling in 14% each [30]. It is still possible that a few additional children with mild disease were missed in this cohort. Similar findings are echoed in a retrospective case series from India [31], where precocious puberty and growth failure were reported in most children. CAH is the most common cause of female ambiguity which presents during adolescence [14,16]. The pubertal changes and advanced skeletal age are irreversible, thus underscoring the need of NBS for timely detection and management of affected children.

In a cohort study at British Columbia Children's Hospital, the median age at diagnosis was 5 days (range, 0–30 days) and 6 days (range, 0–13 days) in unscreened and screened neonates, respectively. However, the cost of care was USD 33,770 per case in unscreened vs. USD 17,726 in screened newborns emphasizing the cost-effectiveness of CAH-NBS program [32]. A cost-benefit analysis is currently not available from India.

Table 1. Published literature on newborn screening for CAH in India.

Author	Year of Publication	Number of Babies Screened	Results	Method Used	False Positivity	Incidence of CAH
Kommalur et al. [33]	2019	41,027	13 babies screen positive, out of which 11 babies could be recalled	17-OHP level by time resolved fluoroimmunoassay	1/11 (9%)	1 in 4102
Verma et al. [34]	2019	13,376	15 babies screen positive; All 15 recalled, 5 found to be true positive	17-OHP level by time resolved fluoroimmunoassay	10/15 (66.7%) were false positive	1 in 2500
ICMR Task force [22]	2018	104,066	142 positive on initial screening; 80% babies could be recalled; 18 infants were confirmed to have CAH (16 salt wasting and 2 simple virilizing)	17-OHP level by time resolved fluoroimmunoassay	96/114 (84.2%) babies false positive	1 in 5762
Anandi et al. [7]	2017	3080 (retrospective analysis)	Retesting done in 82 babies as 17-OHP levels were above cut-off	17-OHP level by competitive enzyme immuno assay	82/82 (100%) babies false positive	-
Kumar et al. [23]	2015	11,200	15 positive on initial screening.	17-OHP level by time resolved fluoroimmunoassay	11/15 (73.3%) babies were false positive	1 in 2800
Kaur et al. [4]	2010	6813	22 positive on initial screening; 7/22 babies could not be recalled;	17-OHP level by time resolved fluoroimmunoassay	13/14 (92.8%) babies false positive	1 in 6813

3. Challenges

3.1. NBS—Current Situation in India

In India, 10% of deliveries are attended by untrained health personnel and only one-third of babies receive a health check-up by trained health-personnel within two days after birth [35]. There is lack of human resource with expertise in childcare and infrastructure for managing sick babies, which, coupled with above observations greatly increase the odds of missing SW and SV-CAH affected babies. Health is a state subject in India which implies that the budget, human resource, logistics and microplanning of any NBS program has to be decentralized and mapped for each state. The current allocation of budget for health in India is also dismal at a meager 1.15% of GDP [36].

As 17OHP levels vary significantly with gestational age, the cut-offs for NBS should be gestational age-specific. However, this may be a concern in cases where pregnancy may be unrecorded and accurate estimation of gestational age is unavailable. The very high proportion of pregnant Indian women with little antenatal care, and that birth weight of Indian babies tend to be lesser than the Western babies for comparable gestational age, underscore the need of local birth weight-based cutoffs. In such situation, birth weight-based cut-offs for 17OHP may be used based on recently compiled data from Indian cohort [5]. Similar weight-based cutoffs were being used in few European countries and Japan [25].

Gender assignment in India is performed immediately after the birth of a baby. This is a major concern for families with the birth of a virilized baby where male gender becomes the default gender within the patriarchal Indian culture. A study from southern India reported incorrect gender assignment in 6/24 (25%) girls, which was correctly reassigned in 5 babies within 1 month of birth, but at six years in the sixth patient [37]. A large dataset of 62 affected CAH patients (6 males) showed ambiguity in 56 (90%), with wrong gender assignment in five affected females [20].

Limited access to specialty endocrinology services and non-availability of appropriate treatment and follow-up facilities remain additional challenges for the babies with CAH, especially from the rural and remote areas. Hydrocortisone, being the drug of choice, has limited availability in remote parts of India, where patients may resort to use of alternative agents like prednisolone or dexamethasone. Chandigarh began newborn screening for CAH for all institutional deliveries in 2007, one of the first states in India to do so [4]. However, the recall and false positive rates were reported to be high in this state, similar to other Asian countries [4,38]. The 'recall rate' means the proportion of babies who the program is able to recall for review following a positive screen, as shown in Table 1. The factors that contribute to poor response to recall include illiteracy, limited healthcare delivery in outreach areas and unawareness of the need for repeating NBS tests. Comprehensive newborn screening is being offered to all births in Kerala, a state in southern India. The NBS program launched in Kerala in 2012, screens for four disorders including congenital hypothyroidism, CAH, Glucose 6 phosphate dehydrogenase deficiency and Galactosemia. Since then, the program has grown to screen more than 140,000 births per year in over 90 government hospitals of Kerala [39].

The lack of NBS across India, even for congenital hypothyroidism, which is a disorder that most developing programs would start with, underscores the need for increasing awareness about the utility of newborn screening in the Indian population. There is also limited public awareness in India about the need to test apparently healthy newborns for life-endangering congenital disorders like CAH. A funded publicity program with contributions from all healthcare professionals (pediatricians, midwives, obstetricians, geneticists and others) will be needed to create this awareness and subsequent agreement to testing and follow up. NBS will have to be eventually integrated with existent maternal and child health programs to ensure universal coverage. Medical colleges and tertiary level hospitals can take the lead in offering NBS services which will later expand their services to cover outreach areas [36].

3.2. Communicating with Families

A diagnosis of CAH is a lifelong identification which should be communicated to the family in a responsive manner. The communication should be done in a more sensitive manner with parents of affected female babies who presented with virilization. The correct gender of the baby should be communicated to the parents ensuring that privacy is maintained. The family is also counseled to maintain confidentiality of the diagnosis to decrease the likely risk of the baby being taken away by eunuch (*hijra*) groups, which are communities of transgender individuals, who are usually considered as social outcastes. This community not only lacks gender recognition and sexual expression, but also has to face limited employment, poor living conditions as well as discrimination on various fronts.

Screening of other members in the family should be performed through a detailed history including three generation pedigree especially in countries which have a high number of consanguineous marriages. In a study from Syria, 14.6% of affected cases had positive family history with a family history of similar complaint in another 18% [40]. An estimated 1–30% marriages are consanguineous in India across different communities [20,41]. Added to this, is the burden of endogamity which increases the probability of manifestation of genetic disorders.

3.3. Healthcare Services (Including Patient Education and Support Groups) in India

There exists an inequitable distribution of healthcare services in India with marked geographical variations which limit access to tertiary level health care services in some areas. The doctor to patient ratio is poor due to the lack of trained and qualified doctors. Thus, the parents of affected children should be educated about adrenal insufficiency and possible risk of adrenal crisis. They should be educated to identify an acute illness at home and increase the dose of replacement steroids to prevent adrenal crisis. An identity card should be carried by all CAH-affected children which should mention the identification details, diagnosis of the child and emergency contact numbers. The card can also mention the need for stress doses of steroids in acute illness which can help in acute management of the child in the remotest corner of the country. The Indian Society for Pediatric and Adolescent Endocrinology (ISPAE) has developed a patient education booklet in English and Hindi (local language) [42]. A similar booklet has been developed by Department of Science and Technology, India in local language (Hindi) for improving patient information. These booklets are shared with the parents at diagnosis which helps them to understand the nature of disease and cope with the stress.

4. Opportunities

The National Health Policy of India, 2017, promotes the provision of quality health care with dynamic cooperation between national and international partners and emphasizes promoting preventive health care, early detection and management of childhood problems [43]. Universal newborn screening for treatable genetic disorders including congenital hypothyroidism and congenital adrenal hyperplasia, however, has still not seen the light of the day in India. Newborn screening in India is only done in a project mode, in specific medical facilities, cities or states, intermittently. The known roadblocks include lack of awareness among healthcare providers, non-institutional deliveries in a significant proportion (22%) of women, logistic and financial issues to cater to a huge birth cohort of 4 million babies annually, lack of sensitization among policy makers and governance issues. To promote the early detection and management of childhood disorders, the Government of India launched the Rashtriya Bal Suraksha Karyakram (RBSK) in 2013, which aimed to screen over 270 million children from 0 to 18 years for four Ds—Defects at birth, Diseases, Deficiencies, and Development Delays including Disabilities. The Delhi government recently launched its flagship health program under the vision of RBSK called 'Mission NEEV' (Neonatal Early Evaluation Vision), to provide universal newborn screening for congenital hypothyroidism and congenital adrenal hyperplasia, early diagnosis of visible birth defects, critical congenital heart diseases and hearing loss. The program is being launched at 31 major birthing facilities of the city and will later be expanded to all delivery points and other birthing facilities [44]. In addition to universal NBS for CAH, it is also important to ensure the appropriate management and long term follow-up of individuals diagnosed with CAH. The potential for working with international partners and funding agencies to establish screening, increase awareness about the need of screening for CAH, patient group advocacy with politicians, starting screening even in small hospitals with patients who can afford additional testing, establishing a dried blood spot diagnostic service for patients at risk capacity building, and dried blood spot technology development in hospitals where this does not exist but which might offer screening in the future, all offer exciting future possibilities. The dried blood spot service can also be used for the monitoring of serial samples in individuals with CAH.

5. Conclusions

NBS offers us hope for the timely detection of CAH. It will help in the timely instituting of therapy to prevent medical and psychosocial complications to improve disease outcomes and decrease the associated morbidity. The logistics for NBS-CAH are limited at present in the Indian context, primarily because of a lack of resources for newborn screening generally, but also because of the limited opportunities to reduce false positive tests by steroid profiling. However, considering not only the mortality and morbidity of severe CAH but also the sizeable population of this treatable condition in India, CAH may be an essential disorder to be screened and included in the core panel of NBS as this is introduced.

Funding: This research received no external funding.

Acknowledgments: We thank B. K. Thelma along with Science and Engineering Board, Department of Science and Technology who helped us in the pilot program for Delhi which has helped us in formulating a program for Delhi now called as MISSION NEEV (Neonatal Early Evaluation Vision).

Conflicts of Interest: The authors declare no conflict of interest.

References

1. Puar, T.H.; Stikkelbroeck, N.M.; Smans, L.C.; Zelissen, P.M.; Hermus, A.R. Adrenal Crisis: Still a Deadly Event in the 21st Century. *Am. J. Med.* **2016**, *129*, 339.e1–339.e9. [CrossRef] [PubMed]
2. Clayton, P.E.; Miller, W.L.; Oberfield, S.E.; Ritzén, E.M.; Sippell, W.G.; Speiser, P.W.; ESPE/LWPES CAH Working Group. Consensus statement on 21-hydroxylase deficiency from the European Society for Paediatric Endocrinology and the Lawson Wilkins Pediatric Endocrine Society. *Horm. Res.* **2002**, *58*, 188–195.
3. Speiser, P.W.; Arlt, W.; Auchus, R.J.; Baskin, L.S.; Conway, G.S.; Merke, D.P.; Meyer-Bahlburg, H.F.; Miller, W.L.; Montori, V.M.; Oberfield, S.E.; et al. Congenital Adrenal Hyperplasia Due to Steroid 21-Hydroxylase Deficiency: An Endocrine Society Clinical Practice Guideline. *J. Clin. Endocrinol. Metab.* **2018**, *103*, 4043–4088. [CrossRef] [PubMed]
4. Kaur, G.; Srivastav, J.; Jain, S.; Chawla, D.; Chavan, B.S.; Atwal, R.; Randhawa, G.; Kaur, A.; Prasad, R. Preliminary report on neonatal screening for congenital hypothyroidism, congenital adrenal hyperplasia and glucose-6-phosphate dehydrogenase deficiency: A Chandigarh experience. *Indian J. Pediatrics* **2010**, *77*, 969–973. [CrossRef] [PubMed]
5. Vats, P.; Dabas, A.; Jain, V.; Seth, A.; Yadav, S.; Kabra, M.; Gupta, N.; Singh, P.; Sharma, R.; Kumar, R.; et al. Newborn Screening and Diagnosis of Infants with Congenital Adrenal Hyperplasia. *Indian Pediatrics* **2020**, *57*, 49–55. [CrossRef] [PubMed]
6. Hall, K. Suitable Specimen Types for Newborn Biochemical Screening-A Summary. *Int. J. Neonatal Screen.* **2017**, *3*, 17. [CrossRef]
7. Anandi, V.S.; Bhattacharya, S. Evaluation of factors associated with elevated newborn 17-hydroxyprogesterone levels. *J. Pediatrics Endocrinol. Metab.* **2017**, *30*, 677–681. [CrossRef] [PubMed]
8. Pearce, M.; Dauerer, E.; DiRienzo, A.G.; Caggana, M.; Tavakoli, N.P. The Influence of Seasonality and Manufacturer Kit Lot Changes on 17α-hydroxyprogesterone Measurements and Referral Rates of Congenital Adrenal Hyperplasia in Newborns. *Eur. J. Pediatrics* **2017**, *176*, 121–129. [CrossRef]

9. González, E.C.; Carvajal, F.; Frómeta, A.; Arteaga, A.L.; Castells, E.M.; Espinosa, T.; Coto, R.; Pérez, P.L.; Tejeda, Y.; Del Río, L.; et al. Newborn screening for congenital adrenal hyperplasia in Cuba: Six years of experience. *Clin. Chim. Acta* **2013**, *421*, 73–78. [CrossRef]
10. Chennuri, V.S.; Mithbawkar, S.M.; Mokal, R.A.; Desai, M.P. Serum 17 alpha hydroxyprogesterone in normal full term and preterm vs sickpreterm and full term newborns in a tertiary hospital. *Indian J. Pediatrics* **2013**, *80*, 21–25. [CrossRef]
11. Number of Births by Type in INDIA FY. 2015–2020. Available online: https://www.statista.com/statistics/659283/childbirths-by-type-india/ (accessed on 7 July 2020).
12. Olgemöller, B.; Roscher, A.A.; Liebl, B.; Fingerhut, R. Screening for congenital adrenal hyperplasia: Adjustment of 17-hydroxyprogesterone cut-off values to both age and birth weight markedly improves the predictive value. *J. Clin. Endocrinol. Metab.* **2003**, *88*, 5790–5794. [CrossRef]
13. Bialk, E.R.; Lasarev, M.R.; Held, P.K. Wisconsin's Screening Algorithm for the identification of Newborns with Congenital Adrenal Hyperplasia. *Int. J. Neonatal Screen.* **2019**, *5*, 33. [CrossRef]
14. Belinda, G.; Vinay, D.; Moolechery, J.; Mathew, V.; Anantharaman, R.; Ayyar, V.; Bantwal, G. Congenital adrenal hyperplasia - experience from a tertiary centre in South India. *Indian J. Endocrinol. Metab.* **2012**, *16*, S385–S386.
15. Walia, R.; Singla, M.; Vaiphei, K.; Kumar, S.; Bhansali, A. Disorders of sex development: A study of 194 cases. *Endocr. Connect.* **2018**, *7*, 364–371. [CrossRef]
16. Misgar, R.A.; Bhat, M.H.; Masoodi, S.R.; Bashir, M.I.; Wani, A.I.; Baba, A.A.; Mufti, G.N.; Bhat, N.A. Disorders of Sex Development: A 10 Years Experience with 73 Cases from the Kashmir Valley. *Indian J. Endocrinol. Metab.* **2019**, *23*, 575–579. [CrossRef]
17. Khan, U.; Lakhani, O.J. Management of primary adrenal insufficiency: Review of current clinical practice in a developed and a developing country. *Indian J. Endocrinol. Metab.* **2017**, *21*, 781–783.
18. Dubey, S.; Tardy, V.; Chowdhury, M.R.; Gupta, N.; Jain, V.; Deka, D.; Sharma, P.; Morel, Y.; Kabra, M. Prenatal diagnosis of steroid 21-hydroxylase-deficient congenital adrenal hyperplasia: Experience from a tertiary care centre in India. *Indian J. Med. Res.* **2017**, *145*, 194–202.
19. Rajendran, U.D.; Kamalarathna, C. Clinical Profile, Predictors of Death andAnthropometric Follow up in Neonateswith Classical 21-Hydroxylase Deficiency. *J. Clin. Diagn. Res.* **2018**, *12*, SC06–SC09.
20. Miati, A.; Chatterjee, S. Congenital adrenal hyperplasia: An Indian experience. *J. Paediatr. Child. Health* **2011**, *47*, 883–887. [CrossRef] [PubMed]
21. Dar, S.A.; Nazir, M.; Lone, R.; Sameen, D.; Ahmad, I.; Wani, W.A.; Charoo, B.A. Clinical Spectrum of Disorders of Sex Development: A Cross-sectional Observational Study. *Indian J. Endocrinol. Metab.* **2018**, *22*, 774–779. [PubMed]
22. Wilson, J.M.G.; Jungner, G. *Principles and Practices of Screening for Disease*; World Health Organization: Geneva, Switzerland, 1968.
23. ICMR Task Force on Inherited Metabolic Disorders. Newborn Screening for Congenital Hypothyroidism and Congenital Adrenal Hyperplasia. *Indian J. Pediatr.* **2018**, *85*, 935–940. [CrossRef] [PubMed]
24. Kumar, R.A.; Das, H.; Kini, P. Newborn screening for congenital adrenal hyperplasia in India: What do we need to watch out for? *J. Obs. Gynaecol. India.* **2016**, *66*, 415–419. [CrossRef] [PubMed]
25. Van der Kamp, H.J.; Wit, J.M. Neonatal screening for congenital adrenal hyperplasia. *Eur. J. Endocrinol.* **2004**, *151*, U71–U75. [CrossRef]
26. Devi, A.R.; Rao, A.N.; Bittles, A.H. Inbreeding and the incidence of childhood genetic disorders in Karnataka, South India. *J. Med. Genet.* **1987**, *24*, 362–365. [CrossRef]
27. Joseph, A.A.; Kulshreshtha, B.; Shabir, I.; Marumudi, E.; George, T.S.; Sagar, R.; Mehta, M.; Ammini, A.C. Gender Issues and Related Social Stigma Affecting Patients with a Disorder of Sex Development in India. *Arch. Sex. Behav.* **2017**, *46*, 361–367. [CrossRef]
28. Speiser, P.W.; Azziz, R.; Baskin, L.S.; Ghizzoni, L.; Hensle, T.W.; Merke, D.P.; Meyer-Bahlburg, H.F.; Miller, W.L.; Montori, V.M.; Oberfield, S.E.; et al. Congenital Adrenal Hyperplasia Due to Steroid 21-Hydroxylase Deficiency: An Endocrine Society Clinical Practice Guideline. *J. Clin. Endocrinol. Metab.* **2010**, *95*, 4133–4160. [CrossRef] [PubMed]
29. Meena, H.; Jana, M.; Singh, V.; Kabra, M.; Jain, V. Growth pattern and clinical profile of Indian children with classical 21-hydroxylase deficiency congenital adrenal hyperplasia on treatment. *Indian J. Pediatr.* **2019**, *86*, 496–502. [CrossRef]

30. Knowles, R.L.; Khalid, J.M.; Oerton, J.M.; Hindmarsh, P.C.; Kelnar, C.J.; Dezateux, C. Late clinical presentation of congenital adrenal hyperplasia in older children: Findings from national paediatric surveillance. *Arch. Dis. Child.* **2014**, *99*, 30–34. [CrossRef]
31. Maheshwari, A.; Khadilkar, V.; Gangodkar, P.; Khadilkar, A. Long-term Growth in Congenital Adrenal Hyperplasia. *Indian J. Pediatr.* **2018**, *85*, 1141–1142. [CrossRef]
32. Fox, D.A.; Ronsley, R.; Khowaja, A.R.; Haim, A.; Vallance, H.; Sinclair, G.; Amed, S. Clinical Impact and Cost Efficacy of Newborn Screening for Congenital Adrenal Hyperplasia. *J. Pediatr.* **2020**, *220*, 101–108. [CrossRef]
33. Kommalur, A.; Devadas, S.; Kariyappa, M.; Sabapathy, S.; Benakappa, A.; Gagandeep, V.; Veranna Sajjan, S.; Krishnapura Lakshminarayana, S.; Dakshayani, B.; Devi Chinnappa, G. Newborn Screening for Five Conditions in a Tertiary Care Government Hospital in Bengaluru, South India—Three Years Experience. *J. Trop. Pediatr.* **2020**, *66*, 284–289. [CrossRef] [PubMed]
34. Verma, J.; Roy, P.; Thomas, D.C.; Jhingan, G.; Singh, A.; Bijarnia-Mahay, S.; Verma, I.C. Newborn Screening for Congenital Hypothyroidism, Congenital Adrenal Hyperplasia, and Glucose-6-Phosphate Dehydrogenase Deficiency for Improving Health Care in India. *J. Pediatr. Intensive Care* **2020**, *9*, 40–44. [CrossRef] [PubMed]
35. Gangaher, A.; Jyotsna, V.P.; Chauhan, V.; John, J.; Mehta, M. Gender of rearing and psychosocial aspect in 46 XX congenital adrenal hyperplasia. *Indian J. Endocrinol. Metab.* **2016**, *20*, 870–877. [PubMed]
36. Kapoor, S.; Gupta, N.; Kabra, M. National newborn screening program—Still a hype or a hope now? *Indian Pediatr.* **2013**, *50*, 639–643. [CrossRef] [PubMed]
37. Bhaskaran, S.; Nair, V.; Kumar, H.; Jayakumar, R.V. Audit of care of patients with congenital adrenal hyperplasia due to 21-Hydroxylase deficiency in a referral hospital in South India. *Indian Pediatr.* **2006**, *43*, 419–423. [PubMed]
38. Amar, H.S.S. Screening for congenital hypothyroidism in Southeast Asia. *J. Paediatr. Obs. Gynaecol.* **1997**, *1*, 5–9.
39. Mookken, T. Universal Implementation of Newborn Screening in India. *Int. J. Neonatal Screen.* **2020**, *6*, 24. [CrossRef]
40. Sheikh Alshabab, L.I.; AlebrahIm, A.; Kaddoura, A.; Al-Fahoum, S. Congenital adrenal hyperplasia due to 21-hydroxylase deficiency: A five-year retrospective study in the Children's Hospital of Damascus, Syria. *Qatar Med. J.* **2015**, *2015*, 11. [CrossRef]
41. Bittles, A. Endogamy, consanguinity and community genetics. *J. Genet.* **2003**, *81*, 91–98. [CrossRef]
42. Indian Society of Pediatric and Adolescent Endocrinology. Patient Resource Congenital Adrenal Hyperplasia. Available online: https://www.ispae.org.in/CAH.php (accessed on 23 January 2020).
43. Ministry of Health and Family Welfare, Government of India. National Health Policy. 2017. Available online: https://mohfw.gov.in/sites/default/files/9147562941489753121.pdf (accessed on 23 January 2020).
44. Delhi Govt Starts 'Mission NEEV' for Early Treatment of Infants. Available online: https://ehealth.eletsonline.com/2020/01/delhi-govt-starts-mission-neev-for-early-treatment-of-infants/ (accessed on 12 February 2020).

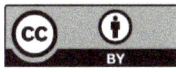

© 2020 by the authors. Licensee MDPI, Basel, Switzerland. This article is an open access article distributed under the terms and conditions of the Creative Commons Attribution (CC BY) license (http://creativecommons.org/licenses/by/4.0/).

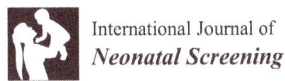

Review

The Success of a Screening Program Is Largely Dependent on Close Collaboration between the Laboratory and the Clinical Follow-Up of the Patients

Svetlana Lajic [1,2], Leif Karlsson [1,3], Rolf H. Zetterström [3,4], Henrik Falhammar [4,5] and Anna Nordenström [1,2,3,*]

1. Department of Women's and Children's Health, Karolinska Institutet, SE-17176 Stockholm, Sweden; Svetlana.Lajic@ki.se (S.L.); Leif.Karlsson@ki.se (L.K.)
2. Pediatric Endocrinology Unit, Astrid Lindgren Children's Hospital, Karolinska University Hospital, SE-17176 Stockholm, Sweden
3. Center for Inherited Metabolic Diseases, Karolinska University Hospital, SE-17176 Stockholm, Sweden; Rolf.Zetterstrom@ki.se
4. Department of Molecular Medicine and Surgery, Karolinska Institutet, SE-17176 Stockholm, Sweden; Henrik.Falhammar@ki.se
5. Department of Endocrinology, Metabolism and Diabetes, Karolinska University Hospital, SE-17176 Stockholm, Sweden
* Correspondence: Anna.Nordenstrom@ki.se; Tel.: +46-85-177-0000

Received: 15 July 2020; Accepted: 24 August 2020; Published: 26 August 2020

Abstract: Neonatal screening for congenital adrenal hyperplasia due to 21-hydroxylase deficiency is now performed in an increasing number of countries all over the world. The main goal of the screening is to achieve early diagnosis and treatment in order to prevent neonatal salt-crisis and death. The screening laboratory can also play an important role in increasing the general awareness of the disease and act as the source of information and education for clinicians to facilitate improved initial care, ensure prompt and correct glucocorticoid dosing to optimize the long-term outcome for the patients. A National CAH Registry and *CYP21A2* genotyping provide valuable information both for evaluating the screening program and the clinical outcome. The Swedish experience is described.

Keywords: neonatal screening; congenital adrenal hyperplasia; CAH; 21-hydroxylase deficiency; long-term outcome

---

1. Introduction

Congenital adrenal hyperplasia (CAH) due to 21-hydroxylase deficiency (21OHD) results in cortisol and aldosterone deficiency. The compensatory increase in ACTH production and concomitant androgen excess is present already in utero and results in virilization of external genitalia in fetuses with a 46, XX karyotype [1]. Before neonatal screening was implemented there was a marked female preponderance among patients with CAH since boys with CAH were diagnosed less often due to a lack of obvious clinical symptoms prior to developing a life-threating salt-losing adrenal crisis in the neonatal period [2]. Lifelong treatment with replacement doses of glucocorticoids and fludrocortisone is required, and during the first year of life additional sodium chloride [1]. Neonatal screening for CAH is now performed in an increasing number of countries throughout the world [3]. The screening was initiated in Sweden in 1986 [4]. The main goal of the screening program is to prevent adrenal salt-crisis and death in the neonatal period [5]. As a secondary benefit, children with less severe forms of CAH diagnosed early may escape early androgen symptoms and instead achieve normal growth and development. The care of individuals with CAH has developed over the past 50 years and the focus is nowadays not only on identification and diagnosis to save lives but the aim is also to improve long-term outcomes and quality of life for the patients [6].

The combination of an efficient neonatal screening program and an optimal treatment and follow-up is key to achieving best possible long-term patient outcomes. Here we describe the Swedish experience and the outcomes and benefit of a close collaboration between the screening laboratory, clinical care, and follow-up.

1.1. Screening

There is one national screening laboratory in Sweden managing more than 100,000 samples per year. Newborn screening is not mandatory in Sweden, but virtually all newborns are screened. The families are given written information at the time the sample is collected and an opt out procedure is employed. Since 2010, the filter paper samples have been collected as soon as possible after 48 h, but were previously collected on day 3–5 [5]. The concentration of 17-hydroxyprogesterone (17OHP) is measured using Genetic Screening Processor (GSP) instruments (Perkin Elmer, Waltham, MA, USA). Gestational age related cut-off levels are used. The cut-off levels have been gradually adjusted over time. At present the cut-off level for full term infants born in or after gestational week (GW) 37 is 60 nmol/L (assuming a hematocrit of 50% in the blood samples). Infants born in GW 35–36 have a cut-off level of 100 nmol/L, and preterm babies born in or before GW 34 have a cut-off level of 350 nmol/L [7].

1.2. Genetics

The genotype-phenotype correlation for 21OHD is well described [8]. Although more than 200 different mutations have been identified today, there is a limited number of mutations that make up more than 90% of the alleles described in patients worldwide [9]. The patients can be divided into four genotype groups based on the severity of the milder allele in compound heterozygous patients: null, I2 splice, I172N, and non-classic CAH. Generally, the null and I2 splice groups are associated with the SW phenotype, I172N with SV CAH, and V281L with NC CAH. P30L results in a phenotype between SV and NC, but was in this study defined as non-classical. A detailed description of all the different mutations in the Swedish cohort has been described elsewhere [6].

2. Short Term Perspective

2.1. Clinical Investigation and Diagnostic Work Up

All screening results above the cut-off level are considered positive screening results [5]. A physician at the laboratory calls out the result to a pediatrician in charge at the local hospital where the child was born, or in the case of preterm infants, to the neonatal ward where the child is presently cared for (see Figure 1). The local physician in charge can thereby receive information about required investigations and treatment and ask questions. The level of 17OHP gives important prognostic information [10]. Advice regarding the dose of hydrocortisone, fludrocortisone, and the likelihood of developing an adrenal salt-crisis and whether the child will require additional sodium chloride can be given. When the level of 17OHP in the screening sample is high and the child is suspected to have the salt wasting form of CAH [10], the urgency is stressed and clinical advice is given about treatment. Consideration of screening 17OHP levels is an important step which provides the opportunity to give detailed recommendations on which additional blood samples to take and whether treatment should be started immediately. Information can be individually tailored to the suspected severity of disease for the specific child. Equally important is the information that a child with a moderately elevated 17OHP, and hence a low risk of salt-loss, can be called in for less urgent assessment the following day. Treatment should in those cases await the results of the follow-up blood tests unless the child has developed symptoms.

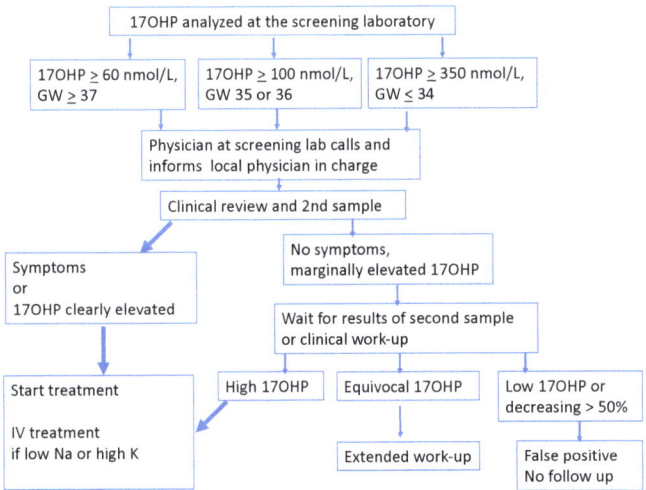

Figure 1. Flow chart for the neonatal screening, 17OHP cut-off levels, information, and investigations.

It is not uncommon that the child is already admitted to the hospital or followed-up because of weight loss or insufficient weight gain when the result of the screening is ready. Hypoglycemia during the first few days of life may also be information that strengthens the suspicion of CAH. The initial symptoms to look for in the neonate with a positive screening test are insufficient weight gain, vomiting, lethargy, hyperpigmentation, clitoral enlargement/penis size, presence or absence of palpable testes, and increased anogenital distance. Analysis of electrolytes, 17OHP, cortisol, a second screening sample on a filter paper card and possibly other hormone analyses depending on the clinical symptoms should be performed. *CYP21A2* mutation analysis gives important prognostic information regarding disease severity and is also informative in investigations of cases where the biochemical diagnostics continue to be unclear.

In cases when the sex of the child is unclear the screening laboratory can perform the screening analysis of 17OHP earlier than at 48 h, and thereby sometimes shorten the time to diagnosis.

2.2. Medical Treatment

The initial hydrocortisone dose given to the child with a newly detected SW form has to be adjusted depending on the clinical situation. If the child has elevated potassium and decreased sodium, treatment should start immediately. Intravenous glucose infusion containing sodium and intravenous hydrocortisone should be given promptly. The initial hydrocortisone bolus dose of 5 mg/kg is followed by 25 mg per 24 h, as a continuous infusion or divided in 3 or 4 doses in our center. The difficulty is often to evaluate if a child is clinically affected when the electrolytes are within the normal range. Our advice, if the diagnosis is likely, considering the level of 17OHP and other clinical symptoms, is to start the treatment with 5 mg × 3 of hydrocortisone orally or intravenously for 2–3 days and then taper down to 2.5 mg × 3 and finally 1 mg × 3. Addition of fludrocortisone and sodium chloride can be given orally if the 17OHP level in the screening is clearly elevated or when the clinical picture is clear and the parents have learned how to give the medication. It may be as important not to over-treat as to avoid an adrenal salt-crises also in the neonatal period.

The *CYP21A2* genotype is determined for virtually all patients in Sweden. The genotype-phenotype correlation for 21OHD is good and genotyping therefore gives valuable support in treatment decisions. Genotyping is also helpful in unclear cases for whom NC CAH may be suspected. However, not all individuals with NC CAH will benefit from starting treatment early [11]. Once a patient is on continuous replacement therapy, it will lead to a decrease in the endogenous glucocorticoid and mineralocorticoid synthesis and put the patient at risk of salt-crises in the event of a stressful situation [11].

3. Long-Term Follow-Up and Perspective

Evaluation of the outcome of the screening program, positive predictive value (PPV) and sensitivity, as well as the outcome for the patients requires follow-up of all patients diagnosed via the screening and patients with a late diagnosis missed by the screening [5]. In Sweden, this is facilitated by the use of a National CAH Registry comprising more than 700 patients today [6]. The severity of CAH among the missed or late diagnosed patients can be determined by *CYP21A2* genotyping. In the registry the *CYP21A2* genotype is known for more than 80% of the patients.

The registry has also made epidemiological studies possible. The patients were anonymized and linked to data of national population-based registers for mortality, somatic, and psychiatric diagnoses in Sweden. One hundred age- and sex-matched controls were selected per patient. In addition, we were able to assess the *CYP21A2* genotype separately (null, I2 splice, I172N, P30L, and NC CAH), as well as outcomes before and after the introduction of the national neonatal screening in 1986.

3.1. Mortality

In two epidemiological studies, one from Sweden and one from the UK, an increased mortality rate was found in patients with CAH (hazard ratio 3–5) with death occurring 6.5–18 years earlier than for controls [12,13]. We were able to show that the neonatal and first year mortality virtually disappeared with the implementation of the neonatal screening for CAH. Interestingly, it was not only the mortality among boys with CAH that was prevented [6]. More girls with the most severe SW form survived with screening, which can be explained by the screening identifying girls who would otherwise have been diagnosed with hypospadias and not have received hydrocortisone treatment. We could also show that the mortality among adults continues to be elevated with a hazard ratio of 2.3–3 in men and women respectively. In almost 50% of the cases the death was related to salt-crises, also among adults. This finding is contradictory to what has been previously generally believed, that the adrenal salt-crises is mainly a risk among children and not a large problem among adults. Next after adrenal crisis, cardiovascular death was the most common cause of death [12] and there was also a documented increased cardiovascular morbidity [14].

3.2. Cardiovascular and Metabolic Risk

Glucocorticoid replacement and androgen control impact the cardiovascular and metabolic risk in patients with CAH [14–16]. Obesity and hypertension, even in young people, may be caused by long-term glucocorticoid replacement [17,18]. Thus, many studies on CAH have suggested an increased cardiovascular and metabolic risk, including insulin resistance [19–21]. However, only occasional studies have been able to show an increased frequency of established cardiovascular disease or diabetes [14,16]. This could be expected since very few studies have included patients with CAH above the age of 50 years when cardiovascular disease and diabetes usually appear. Different genotypes may have different risk for cardiovascular events [14]. In the epidemiological study of the entire Swedish population and in all patients with CAH ($n = 588$) the risk for any cardiometabolic disease, any cardiovascular disease, obesity, diabetes, obstructive sleep apnea, dyslipidemia, hypertension, atrial fibrillation, and venous thromboembolism was significantly increased compared to matched controls ($n = 58,800$) [14]. Cardiovascular and metabolic issues still occurred in those born after the introduction of neonatal screening in 1986 in Sweden, especially any cardiovascular and metabolic disorder, obesity, and hypertension [14]. However, other studies have indicated that a late diagnosis of CAH may be associated with increased cardiometabolic risk [16,20]. Thus, early diagnosis and regular monitoring of cardiometabolic risk in patients with CAH is important.

3.3. Fertility Issues

Fertility has been reported to be impaired in both females and males with CAH [9,22]. In women high androgen and 17OHP concentrations lead to menstrual irregularities and anovulation [1]. Continuous high progesterone concentrations result in a contraceptive effect, but optimizing glucocorticoid replacement can normalize the hormonal situation and improve fertility [23]. However, decreased sexual activity, higher sexual distress, higher prevalence of homosexuality or bisexuality, and disinterest in pursuing motherhood most likely play a role in the decreased fertility rate [24,25]. Those with a more severe genotype/phenotype have a lower fertility rate [22,24]. Fertility in males with CAH is impaired [26,27], mainly due to hyper- or hypogonadotropic hypogonadism and testicular adrenal rest tumors (TARTs) [28]. These tumors were reported in up to 86% of all adult males with CAH [29]. In the Swedish epidemiological study including 221 males with CAH only those born before the neonatal screening had impaired fertility while those born after the introduction of screening had normalized fertility compared to same age controls [27]. One can speculate if the mini-puberty or an imbalance in FSH, LH, and gonadal synthesis of testosterone or other steroid hormones during the first year of life may be of importance [30]. It is unclear if the same is true for females with CAH but fertility rates have improved over the years and may now slowly approach that of the general population [31]. If the improved fertility is due to better and individualized fertility therapy, better general management of CAH or the introduction of neonatal screening is unclear. Thus, early diagnosis may improve fertility, at least in males with CAH.

3.4. Stress Vulnerability and Psychiatric Diagnoses

Stress vulnerability seems to be increased in patients with CAH and has been suggested to be one of the causes of increased sick leave and disability pension in CAH compared to matched controls [22]. Only a few investigations on psychiatric diagnosis in CAH have been reported. Psychiatric diseases seem more common [13,16,32,33], especially depression [13,32–34], alcohol misuse [32,33] and suicidality [16,32], which can be interpreted as stress related. Around 10% of the mortality in CAH was caused by suicide [12] but in males with CAH born after the introduction of the neonatal screening no increase in any psychiatric disorder or suicidality were seen [32]. However, in females with CAH a similar over representation in any psychiatric disorder were seen before and after the introduction of the neonatal screening, even though the spectrum of psychiatric diagnosis was slightly different [33]. Females with the null genotype born before the introduction of the neonatal screening were more likely to be diagnosed with ADHD [33]. The explanations may be increased androgen exposure, repeated episodes of hypoglycemia or salt-crises, all more prevalent before the introduction of neonatal screening. Moreover, males diagnosed late had more depressive symptoms and lower self-control compared to controls [35]. Early exposure to elevated androgen levels or supra-physiologic glucocorticoid doses may have secondary effects on the function of the pituitary–adrenal-axis later in life, contributing to stress vulnerability [36]. Hence, a later diagnosis may increase the risk of a psychiatric diagnosis.

3.5. Cognition

It is known that the brain is sensitive to exposure to high levels of cortisol and other glucocorticoids and that it may be more vulnerable early in the development. The treatment in CAH is life long and it is a continuous process to adjust the dose of glucocorticoid throughout childhood and adult life. Worldwide studies have repeatedly shown that individuals with CAH have negatively affected cognition. However, the results from studies investigating cognitive outcome in patients with CAH have been disparate. In some studies, adults with CAH have a lower full-scale IQ compared to controls [37–40], but other studies show a normal general intellectual capacity, irrespective of age [41]. While results differ between studies regarding the full-scale IQ, an observation that seems to be consistent is that patients with CAH often have an impaired working memory performance [42–45].

The effects on working memory were seen as early as during childhood in patients that did not undergo neonatal screening for CAH [43].

Interestingly, in a Swedish cohort of children with CAH, with good metabolic control, that was identified through neonatal screening and treated early with a three- or four-dose regimen with hydrocortisone we could not see any negative impact on executive functioning or memory [46]. This emphasizes the importance of an early diagnosis, before the development of an adrenal crisis, and adequate glucocorticoid dosing and good adherence to therapy [46].

More recent observational studies from the UK, USA, and Sweden regarding brain morphology in patients with CAH have revealed that patients show reductions in cortical and limbic regions of the brain that are important for the working memory [45,47,48]. This new evidence points to the fact that alterations in brain structure and possibly also in the functional organization of the brain may underlie the cognitive changes [45,47,48]. In the UK study [45], patients with CAH showed reductions in volumes of the right hippocampus, left amygdala, bilateral thalamus, cerebellum, and brainstem. The study cohort included only women (age range 18–50 years), most patients were treated with hydrocortisone, and 40% with prednisolone. The majority of the patients had SW CAH and 74% of the patients had a null genotype [45].

The American cohort [48] comprised children (age range 8–18 years) and analyzed the MRI data with a focus on the prefrontal cortex and regions of the hippocampus and the amygdala. The patients almost exclusively had SW CAH and approximately half of the cohort was diagnosed through neonatal screening. Patients were treated either with hydrocortisone, prednisolone, or dexamethasone. Also here, reductions in the volumes of the prefrontal cortex, amygdala, and hippocampus were observed [48].

The Swedish study [47] included both women and men in a large cohort of adolescents and young adults with CAH (age range 16–32 years). Most patients were treated with hydrocortisone and the majority was diagnosed through the Swedish neonatal screening program for CAH. The authors could not identify structural disturbances in limbic structures but changes were observed in the prefrontal, parietal, and superior cortex, regions important for working memory functioning. Interestingly, there was a positive association between the grey matter structures and the nucleus precuneus with working memory performance [47].

Imbalances in hormonal levels such as over- or undertreatment with glucocorticoids or the difficulty in mimicking the circadian and ultradian cortisol rhythm, repeated episodes of hypoglycemia, or salt-losing crises may affect brain structures and the cognitive abilities in patients with CAH [37–40,42–44,46]. Given this, optimal glucocorticoid treatment is a key factor in improving long term cognitive outcomes in patients with CAH.

Neurons within the amygdala, hippocampus, and the prefrontal cortex express both mineralocorticoid receptor and glucocorticoid receptor at high levels, and the glucocorticoid receptor is also widely expressed throughout the brain [49–51]. These areas, important for executive functioning, emotional regulation, and memory [52–54] have been shown to be vulnerable to high levels of glucocorticoids. In addition, the severity of CAH has also been shown to affect the cognitive outcome possibly through differences in androgen exposure, hypoglycemia, salt-losing crises, and differences in treatment regimen [43,44]. The differences in patient outcome most likely is the product of a combination of the previously mentioned factors and the choice of treatment such as type of glucocorticoid [40,45,46].

The vulnerability of the brain in the neonatal period and early in life makes it important to detect the patients as early as possible to avoid adrenal salt-crises, and possibly hypoglycemia before start of treatment. It is possible that, in addition, avoiding treatment with extremely high stress-doses of glucocorticoid in the neonatal period may be an important factor. Early diagnosis and treatment may also be important for psychological factors, vulnerability to stress, and cardiovascular/metabolic morbidity over the course of the lifetime. Close follow-up and adjustment of the replacement doses to mimic the circadian rhythm, avoid salt crises and hypoglycemia, and at the same time avoid overtreatment all through childhood is of course imperative but at times a challenging task.

4. Conclusions

Improvements in the overall outcome for patients with CAH require a close collaboration between the screening laboratory and the clinicians. *CYP21A2* genotyping is instrumental in the follow-up and evaluation of the screening program and gives valuable guidance in the clinical care of the patients. The screening program increases the general awareness of the disease and the knowledge about treatment. The screening lab can also act as the source of information and education for clinicians especially in a large country with a relatively small population like Sweden with few specialized centers. This facilitates improved initial care, ensures prompt and correct glucocorticoid dosing, and avoids overtreatment and its potential negative effects on the brain and development. From the current evidence, it seems that implementation of neonatal screening and avoiding long-acting and high doses of glucocorticoids complemented with a good clinical management over time is key for improving long-term outcome for the patients with CAH.

Author Contributions: Conceptualization A.N. and R.H.Z.; Original Draft Preparation: A.N., H.F., S.L., and L.K.; Writing—review and editing: A.N., H.F., S.L., and R.H.Z.; Supervision: A.N. All authors have read and agreed to the published version of the manuscript.

Funding: This was funded by Stockholm County Council (ALF-SLL) 108223.

Conflicts of Interest: The authors declare no conflict of interest.

References

1. Speiser, P.W.; Arlt, W.; Auchus, R.J.; Baskin, L.S.; Conway, G.S.; Merke, D.P.; Meyer-Bahlburg, H.F.L.; Miller, W.L.; Murad, M.H.; Oberfield, S.E.; et al. Congenital Adrenal Hyperplasia Due to Steroid 21-Hydroxylase Deficiency: An Endocrine Society Clinical Practice Guideline. *J. Clin. Endocrinol. Metab.* **2018**, *103*, 4043–4088. [CrossRef]
2. Nordenstrom, A.; Ahmed, S.; Jones, J.; Coleman, M.; Price, D.A.; Clayton, P.E.; Hall, C.M. Female preponderance in congenital adrenal hyperplasia due to CYP21 deficiency in England: Implications for neonatal screening. *Horm. Res.* **2005**, *63*, 22–28. [CrossRef] [PubMed]
3. White, P.C. Optimizing newborn screening for congenital adrenal hyperplasia. *J. Pediatr.* **2013**, *163*, 10–12. [CrossRef] [PubMed]
4. Thilén, A.; Nordenstrom, A.; Hagenfeldt, L.; von Dobeln, U.; Guthenberg, C.; Larsson, A. Benefits of neonatal screening for congenital adrenal hyperplasia (21-hydroxylase deficiency) in Sweden. *Pediatrics* **1998**, *101*, E11. [CrossRef] [PubMed]
5. Gidlof, S.; Wedell, A.; Guthenberg, C.; von Dobeln, U.; Nordenstrom, A. Nationwide neonatal screening for congenital adrenal hyperplasia in sweden: A 26-year longitudinal prospective population-based study. *JAMA Pediatr.* **2014**, *168*, 567–574. [CrossRef]
6. Gidlöf, S.; Falhammar, H.; Thilén, A.; von Döbeln, A.; Ritzén, M.; Wedell, A.; Nordenström, A. One hundred years of congenital adrenal hyperplasia in Sweden: A retrospective, population-based cohort study. *Lancet Diabetes Endocrinol.* **2013**, *1*, 35–43. [CrossRef]
7. Zetterström, R.; Karlsson, L.; Falhammar, H.; Lajic, S.; Nordenstrom, A. Update on the Swedish Newborn Screening for Congenital Adrenal Hyperplasia due to 21-hydroxylase Deficiency. *Int. J. Neonatal Screen* **2020**, submitted.
8. Krone, N.; Arlt, W. Genetics of congenital adrenal hyperplasia. *Best Pract. Res. Clin. Endocrinol. Metab.* **2009**, *23*, 181–192. [CrossRef]
9. Speiser, P.W.; Azziz, R.; Baskin, L.S.; Ghizzoni, L.; Hensle, T.W.; Merke, D.P.; Meyer-Bahlburg, H.F.; Miller, W.L.; Montori, V.M.; Oberfield, S.E.; et al. Congenital adrenal hyperplasia due to steroid 21-hydroxylase deficiency: An Endocrine Society clinical practice guideline. *J. Clin. Endocrinol. Metab.* **2010**, *95*, 4133–4160. [CrossRef]
10. Nordenstrom, A.; Thilen, A.; Hagenfeldt, L.; Larsson, A.; Wedell, A. Genotyping is a valuable diagnostic complement to neonatal screening for congenital adrenal hyperplasia due to steroid 21-hydroxylase deficiency. *J. Clin. Endocrinol. Metab.* **1999**, *84*, 1505–1509. [CrossRef]

11. Nordenstrom, A.; Falhammar, H. Management of Endocrine Disease: Diagnosis and management of the patient with non-classic CAH due to 21-hydroxylase deficiency. *Eur. J. Endocrinol.* **2019**, *180*, R127–R145. [CrossRef] [PubMed]
12. Falhammar, H.; Frisen, L.; Norrby, C.; Hirschberg, A.L.; Almqvist, C.; Nordenskjold, A.; Nordenstrom, A. Increased mortality in patients with congenital adrenal hyperplasia due to 21-hydroxylase deficiency. *J. Clin. Endocrinol. Metab.* **2014**, *99*, E2715–E2721. [CrossRef] [PubMed]
13. Jenkins-Jones, S.; Parviainen, L.; Porter, J.; Withe, M.; Whitaker, M.J.; Holden, S.E.; Morgan, C.L.; Currie, C.J.; Ross, R.J.M. Poor compliance and increased mortality, depression and healthcare costs in patients with congenital adrenal hyperplasia. *Eur. J. Endocrinol.* **2018**, *178*, 309–320. [CrossRef] [PubMed]
14. Falhammar, H.; Frisen, L.; Hirschberg, A.L.; Norrby, C.; Almqvist, C.; Nordenskjold, A.; Nordenstrom, A. Increased Cardiovascular and Metabolic Morbidity in Patients With 21-Hydroxylase Deficiency: A Swedish Population-Based National Cohort Study. *J. Clin. Endocrinol. Metab.* **2015**, *100*, 3520–3528. [CrossRef]
15. Paizoni, L.; Auer, M.K.; Schmidt, H.; Hubner, A.; Bidlingmaier, M.; Reisch, N. Effect of androgen excess and glucocorticoid exposure on metabolic risk profiles in patients with congenital adrenal hyperplasia due to 21-hydroxylase deficiency. *J. Steroid Biochem. Mol. Biol.* **2020**, *197*, 105540. [CrossRef]
16. Falhammar, H.; van der Claahsen-Grinten, H.; Reisch, N.; Slowikowska-Hilczer, J.; Nordenstrom, A.; Roehle, R.; Bouvattier, C.; Kreukels, B.P.; Kohler, B. Health status in 1040 adults with disorders of sex development (DSD): A European multicenter study. *Endocr. Connect.* **2018**, *7*, 466–478. [CrossRef]
17. Arlt, W.; Willis, D.S.; Wild, S.H.; Krone, N.; Doherty, E.J.; Hahner, S.; Han, T.S.; Carroll, P.V.; Conway, G.S.; Rees, D.A.; et al. Health status of adults with congenital adrenal hyperplasia: A cohort study of 203 patients. *J. Clin. Endocrinol. Metab.* **2010**, *95*, 5110–5121. [CrossRef]
18. Kim, M.S.; Ryabets-Lienhard, A.; Dao-Tran, A.; Mittelman, S.D.; Gilsanz, V.; Schrager, S.M.; Geffner, M.E. Increased Abdominal Adiposity in Adolescents and Young Adults With Classical Congenital Adrenal Hyperplasia due to 21-Hydroxylase Deficiency. *J. Clin. Endocrinol. Metab.* **2015**, *100*, E1153–E1159. [CrossRef]
19. Finkielstain, G.P.; Kim, M.S.; Sinaii, N.; Nishitani, M.; Van Ryzin, C.; Hill, S.C.; Reynolds, J.C.; Hanna, R.M.; Merke, D.P. Clinical characteristics of a cohort of 244 patients with congenital adrenal hyperplasia. *J. Clin. Endocrinol. Metab.* **2012**, *97*, 4429–4438. [CrossRef]
20. Zhang, H.J.; Yang, J.; Zhang, M.N.; Liu, C.Q.; Xu, M.; Li, X.J.; Yang, S.Y.; Li, X.Y. Metabolic disorders in newly diagnosed young adult female patients with simple virilizing 21-hydroxylase deficiency. *Endocrine* **2010**, *38*, 260–265. [CrossRef]
21. Mooij, C.F.; Pourier, M.S.; Weijers, G.; de Korte, C.L.; Fejzic, Z.; Claahsen-van der Grinten, H.L.; Kapusta, L. Cardiac function in paediatric patients with congenital adrenal hyperplasia due to 21 hydroxylase deficiency. *Clin. Endocrinol.* **2018**, *88*, 364–371. [CrossRef] [PubMed]
22. Strandqvist, A.; Falhammar, H.; Lichtenstein, P.; Hirschberg, A.L.; Wedell, A.; Norrby, C.; Nordenskjold, A.; Frisen, L.; Nordenstrom, A. Suboptimal psychosocial outcomes in patients with congenital adrenal hyperplasia: Epidemiological studies in a nonbiased national cohort in Sweden. *J. Clin. Endocrinol. Metab.* **2014**, *99*, 1425–1432. [CrossRef] [PubMed]
23. Reichman, D.E.; White, P.C.; New, M.I.; Rosenwaks, Z. Fertility in patients with congenital adrenal hyperplasia. *Fertil. Steril.* **2014**, *101*, 301–309. [CrossRef] [PubMed]
24. Gomes, L.G.; Bachega, T.; Mendonca, B.B. Classic congenital adrenal hyperplasia and its impact on reproduction. *Fertil. Steril.* **2019**, *111*, 7–12. [CrossRef] [PubMed]
25. Hagenfeldt, K.; Janson, P.O.; Holmdahl, G.; Falhammar, H.; Filipsson, H.; Frisen, L.; Thoren, M.; Nordenskjold, A. Fertility and pregnancy outcome in women with congenital adrenal hyperplasia due to 21-hydroxylase deficiency. *Hum. Reprod.* **2008**, *23*, 1607–1613. [CrossRef]
26. Bouvattier, C.; Esterle, L.; Renoult-Pierre, P.; de la Perriere, A.B.; Illouz, F.; Kerlan, V.; Pascal-Vigneron, V.; Drui, D.; Christin-Maitre, S.; Galland, F.; et al. Clinical Outcome, Hormonal Status, Gonadotrope Axis, and Testicular Function in 219 Adult Men Born With Classic 21-Hydroxylase Deficiency. A French National Survey. *J. Clin. Endocrinol. Metab.* **2015**, *100*, 2303–2313. [CrossRef]
27. Falhammar, H.; Frisen, L.; Norrby, C.; Almqvist, C.; Hirschberg, A.L.; Nordenskjold, A.; Nordenstrom, A. Reduced Frequency of Biological and Increased Frequency of Adopted Children in Males With 21-Hydroxylase Deficiency: A Swedish Population-Based National Cohort Study. *J. Clin. Endocrinol. Metab.* **2017**, *102*, 4191–4199. [CrossRef]

28. Engels, M.; Span, P.N.; van Herwaarden, A.E.; Sweep, F.; Stikkelbroeck, N.; Claahsen-van der Grinten, H.L. Testicular Adrenal Rest Tumors: Current Insights on Prevalence, Characteristics, Origin, and Treatment. *Endocr. Rev.* **2019**, *40*, 973–987. [CrossRef]
29. Falhammar, H.; Nystrom, H.F.; Ekstrom, U.; Granberg, S.; Wedell, A.; Thoren, M. Fertility, sexuality and testicular adrenal rest tumors in adult males with congenital adrenal hyperplasia. *Eur. J. Endocrinol.* **2012**, *166*, 441–449. [CrossRef]
30. Lanciotti, L.; Cofini, M.; Leonardi, A.; Penta, L.; Esposito, S. Up-To-Date Review about Minipuberty and Overview on Hypothalamic-Pituitary-Gonadal Axis Activation in Fetal and Neonatal Life. *Front. Endocrinol.* **2018**, *9*, 410. [CrossRef]
31. Lekarev, O.; Lin-Su, K.; Vogiatzi, M.G. Infertility and Reproductive Function in Patients with Congenital Adrenal Hyperplasia: Pathophysiology, Advances in Management, and Recent Outcomes. *Endocrinol. Metab. Clin. N. Am.* **2015**, *44*, 705–722. [CrossRef]
32. Falhammar, H.; Butwicka, A.; Landen, M.; Lichtenstein, P.; Nordenskjold, A.; Nordenstrom, A.; Frisen, L. Increased psychiatric morbidity in men with congenital adrenal hyperplasia due to 21-hydroxylase deficiency. *J. Clin. Endocrinol. Metab.* **2014**, *99*, E554–E560. [CrossRef]
33. Engberg, H.; Butwicka, A.; Nordenstrom, A.; Hirschberg, A.L.; Falhammar, H.; Lichtenstein, P.; Nordenskjold, A.; Frisen, L.; Landen, M. Congenital adrenal hyperplasia and risk for psychiatric disorders in girls and women born between 1915 and 2010: A total population study. *Psychoneuroendocrinology* **2015**, *60*, 195–205. [CrossRef] [PubMed]
34. Nordenskjold, A.; Holmdahl, G.; Frisen, L.; Falhammar, H.; Filipsson, H.; Thoren, M.; Janson, P.O.; Hagenfeldt, K. Type of mutation and surgical procedure affect long-term quality of life for women with congenital adrenal hyperplasia. *J. Clin. Endocrinol. Metab.* **2008**, *93*, 380–386. [CrossRef] [PubMed]
35. Falhammar, H.; Nystrom, H.F.; Thoren, M. Quality of life, social situation, and sexual satisfaction, in adult males with congenital adrenal hyperplasia. *Endocrine* **2014**, *47*, 299–307. [CrossRef] [PubMed]
36. Gunnar, M.R.; Quevedo, K.M. Early care experiences and HPA axis regulation in children: A mechanism for later trauma vulnerability. *Prog. Brain Res.* **2008**, *167*, 137–149. [CrossRef]
37. Johannsen, T.H.; Ripa, C.P.L.; Reinisch, J.M.; Schwartz, M.; Mortensen, E.L.; Main, K.M. Impaired Cognitive Function in Women with Congenital Adrenal Hyperplasia. *J. Clin. Endocrinol. Metab.* **2006**, *91*, 1376–1381. [CrossRef]
38. Helleday, J.; Bartfai, I.A.; Ritzén, E.M.; Forsman, M. Generel Intelligence and Cognitive Profile in Women with Congenital Adrenal Hyperplasia (CAH). *Psychoneuroendocrinoiogy* **1994**, *19*, 343–356. [CrossRef]
39. Hamed, S.A.; Metwalley, K.A.; Farghaly, H.S. Cognitive function in children with classic congenital adrenal hyperplasia. *Eur. J. Pediatr.* **2018**, *177*, 1633–1640. [CrossRef]
40. Amr, N.H.; Baioumi, A.Y.; Serour, M.N.; Khalifa, A.; Shaker, N.M. Cognitive functions in children with congenital adrenal hyperplasia. *Arch. Endocrinol. Metab.* **2019**, *63*, 113–120. [CrossRef]
41. Berenbaum, S.A.; Bryk, K.K.; Duck, S.C. Normal intelligence in female and male patients with congenital adrenal hyperplasia. *Int. J. Pediatr. Endocrinol.* **2010**, *2010*, 853103. [CrossRef] [PubMed]
42. Collaer, M.L.; Hindmarsh, P.C.; Pasterski, V.; Fane, B.A.; Hines, M. Reduced short term memory in congenital adrenal hyperplasia (CAH) and its relationship to spatial and quantitative performance. *Psychoneuroendocrinology* **2016**, *64*, 164–173. [CrossRef] [PubMed]
43. Browne, W.V.; Hindmarsh, P.C.; Pasterski, V.; Hughes, I.A.; Acerini, C.L.; Spencer, D.; Neufeld, S.; Hines, M. Working memory performance is reduced in children with congenital adrenal hyperplasia. *Horm. Behav.* **2015**, *67*, 83–88. [CrossRef] [PubMed]
44. Karlsson, L.; Gezelius, A.; Nordenstrom, A.; Hirvikoski, T.; Lajic, S. Cognitive impairment in adolescents and adults with congenital adrenal hyperplasia. *Clin. Endocrinol.* **2017**, *87*, 651–659. [CrossRef]
45. Webb, E.A.; Elliott, L.; Carlin, D.; Wilson, M.; Hall, K.; Netherton, J.; Reed, J.; Barrett, T.G.; Salwani, V.; Clayden, J.D.; et al. Quantitative Brain MRI in Congenital Adrenal Hyperplasia: In Vivo Assessment of the Cognitive and Structural Impact of Steroid Hormones. *J. Clin. Endocrinol. Metab.* **2018**, *103*, 1330–1341. [CrossRef]
46. Messina, V.; Karlsson, L.; Hirvikoski, T.; Nordenstrom, A.; Lajic, S. Cognitive Function of Children and Adolescents With Congenital Adrenal Hyperplasia: Importance of Early Diagnosis. *J. Clin. Endocrinol. Metab.* **2020**, *105*, e683–e691. [CrossRef]

47. van't Westeinde, A.; Karlsson, L.; Thomsen Sandberg, M.; Nordenström, A.; Padilla, N.; Lajic, S. Altered Gray Matter Structure and White Matter Microstructure in Patients with Congenital Adrenal Hyperplasia: Relevance for Working Memory Performance. *Cereb. Cortex* **2019**, *30*, 2777–2788. [CrossRef]
48. Herting, M.M.; Azad, A.; Kim, R.; Tyszka, J.M.; Geffner, M.E.; Kim, M.S. Brain Differences in the Prefrontal Cortex, Amygdala, and Hippocampus in Youth with Congenital Adrenal Hyperplasia. *J. Clin. Endocrinol. Metab.* **2020**, *105*, 1098–1111. [CrossRef]
49. Colciago, A.; Casati, L.; Negri-Cesi, P.; Celotti, F. Learning and memory: Steroids and epigenetics. *J. Steroid Biochem. Mol. Biol.* **2015**, *150*, 64–85. [CrossRef]
50. Matsusue, Y.; Horii-Hayashi, N.; Kirita, T.; Nishi, M. Distribution of corticosteroid receptors in mature oligodendrocytes and oligodendrocyte progenitors of the adult mouse brain. *J. Histochem. Cytochem.* **2014**, *62*, 211–226. [CrossRef]
51. de Kloet, E.R.; Joels, M.; Holsboer, F. Stress and the brain: From adaptation to disease. *Nat. Rev. Neurosci.* **2005**, *6*, 463–475. [CrossRef] [PubMed]
52. LeDoux, J.E. Emotion Circuits in the Brain. *Annu. Rev. Neurosci.* **2000**, *23*, 155–184. [CrossRef] [PubMed]
53. Funahashi, S. Neuronal mechanisms of executive control by the prefrontal cortex. *Neurosci. Res.* **2001**, *39*, 147–165. [CrossRef]
54. Opitz, B. Memory Function and the Hippocampus. *Front. Neurol. Neurosci.* **2014**, *34*, 51–59. [CrossRef]

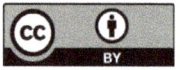

© 2020 by the authors. Licensee MDPI, Basel, Switzerland. This article is an open access article distributed under the terms and conditions of the Creative Commons Attribution (CC BY) license (http://creativecommons.org/licenses/by/4.0/).

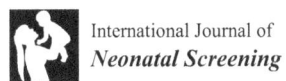

Review

Newborn Screening for Congenital Adrenal Hyperplasia: Review of Factors Affecting Screening Accuracy

Patrice K. Held [1,2,*], Ian M. Bird [3] and Natasha L. Heather [4,5]

1. Wisconsin State Laboratory of Hygiene, University of Wisconsin School of Medicine and Public Health, Madison, WI 53706, USA
2. Department of Pediatrics, University of Wisconsin School of Medicine and Public Health, Madison, WI 53706, USA
3. Department of Obstetrics and Gynecology, University of Wisconsin School of Medicine and Public Health, Madison, WI 53715, USA; imbird@wisc.edu
4. Newborn Screening, LabPlus, Auckland City Hospital, Auckland 1023, New Zealand; NHeather@adhb.govt.nz
5. Liggins Institute, University of Auckland, Auckland 1010, New Zealand
* Correspondence: patrice.held@slh.wisc.edu; Tel.: +1-608-265-5968

Received: 25 June 2020; Accepted: 17 August 2020; Published: 23 August 2020

Abstract: Newborn screening for 21-hydroxylase deficiency (21OHD), the most common form of congenital adrenal hyperplasia, has been performed routinely in the United States and other countries for over 20 years. Screening provides the opportunity for early detection and treatment of patients with 21OHD, preventing salt-wasting crisis during the first weeks of life. However, current first-tier screening methodologies lack specificity, leading to a large number of false positive cases, and adequate sensitivity to detect all cases of classic 21OHD that would benefit from treatment. This review summarizes the pathology of 21OHD and also the key stages of fetal hypothalamic-pituitary-adrenal axis development and adrenal steroidogenesis that contribute to limitations in screening accuracy. Factors leading to both false positive and false negative results are highlighted, along with specimen collection best practices used by laboratories in the United States and worldwide. This comprehensive review provides context and insight into the limitations of newborn screening for 21OHD for laboratorians, primary care physicians, and endocrinologists.

Keywords: congenital adrenal hyperplasia; newborn screening

---

1. Introduction

Congenital adrenal hyperplasia (CAH) refers to a group of inherited genetic disorders caused by specific enzyme defects within the biosynthetic pathway of glucocorticoids. 21-hydroxylase deficiency (21OHD) is the most common cause of CAH, accounting for over 95% of all cases [1].

Newborns with untreated severe 21OHD, referred to as salt-wasting CAH (SW-CAH), develop progressive salt-wasting crisis during the first weeks of life, resulting in significant morbidity and mortality [2]. Newborn screening for SW-CAH provides the opportunity for early detection and treatment and has been implemented in the United States and more than 35 countries [3]. However, at present, first-tier screening methodologies lack specificity and adequate sensitivity to identify all newborns with 21OHD that would benefit from early treatment [1].

Here, we provide an overview of CAH due to 21OHD, focusing on disease presentation, pathology, genetics, diagnosis, and treatment. Next, we review the development stages of the fetal hypothalamic-pituitary-adrenal axis and adrenal steroidogenesis, so that the reader can better understand the biological processes that contribute to false positive and false negative results in newborn screening. Lastly, we will summarize different screening algorithms and approaches to specimen collection used by laboratories in the United States and worldwide to enhance detection of newborns with 21OHD.

2. Features of 21-Hydroxylase Deficiency

2.1. Clinical Manifestations

Patients with 21OHD have a range of clinical presentations which are categorized into three groups: classic salt-wasting (SW-CAH), classic simple-virilizing (SV-CAH), and non-classic (NC-CAH). The combined estimated incidence of classic 21OHD is 1 in 14,000 to 18,000 live births, with approximately 75% classified as SW-CAH and 25% classified as SV-CAH. NC-CAH is more common than the classic forms, with an estimated incidence of 1 in 200 [1].

Patients with the most severe form, SW-CAH, have <2% 21-hydroxylase activity and are unable to produce adequate amounts (if any) of cortisol and aldosterone. A salt-wasting crisis can be evident within the first 5 days of life and is characterized by progressive hyponatremia, hyperkalemia, dehydration, alkalosis, and failure to thrive, leading to shock and ultimately death, if left untreated. Patients with SV-CAH have slightly higher residual enzyme activity, as compared to the SW-CAH patients, and can generally secrete adequate amounts of aldosterone to maintain sodium balance and prevent a salt-wasting crisis [1,4].

Excess adrenal androgen production is an additional feature of 21OHD. Prenatal virilization occurs in both SW-CAH and SV-CAH and can present clinically as ambiguous genitalia in females. However, the degree of genital virilization is variable and detection is reliant on clinical acumen, such that females are at times missed or misidentified as males [5,6]. Males with 21OHD are less readily detected on clinical examination and therefore are more likely to benefit from newborn screening. Of note, data from the Sweden screening program suggests that clinical detection of classic 21OHD may be similarly unreliable for both genders [7]. Males and females with SV-CAH, who are not identified in the neonatal period, typically present in early childhood with premature development of pubic hair and rapid skeletal growth [4].

Patients with NC-CAH have up to 50% of normal 21-hydroxylase activity. The adequate amounts of cortisol and aldosterone production prevent severe clinical deficiencies. Post-natal androgen excess is variable and many patients with NC-CAH remain undiagnosed. Signs of androgen excess during childhood are less obvious and include premature adrenarche, rapid skeletal growth, and cystic acne. Common presenting features for affected adult women include hirsutism, menstrual cycle disorders, and decreased fertility [1,4].

2.2. Pathology

In the adrenal steroidogenic pathway, 21-hydroxylase (P450c21) catalyzes the conversion of 17-hydroxyprogesterone (17OHP) to 11-deoxycortisol to form cortisol and the conversion of progesterone to 11-deoxycorticosterone to form aldosterone (P450c21, in red, Figure 1). The required levels of cortisol (µg/dL, nmol/L range) far exceeds aldosterone (ng/dL, pmol/L range) and thereby the presence of only minimal 21-hydroxylase activity (1–2%) can produce adequate amounts of aldosterone to prevent a salt-wasting crisis [8].

Patients with 21OHD have reduced or absent production of cortisol. This deficiency leads to an uninhibited overproduction of pituitary adrenocorticotropic hormone (ACTH) in an attempt to stimulate adrenal steroidogenesis. Concentrations of steroid precursors, prior to the enzyme block, accumulate in response to this ACTH stimulation. The adrenal steroid precursors, pregnenolone, and 17-hydroxypregnenolone, are sequestered for the biosynthesis and ultimately overproduction of dehydroepiandrosterone (DHEA) and other androgens [4].

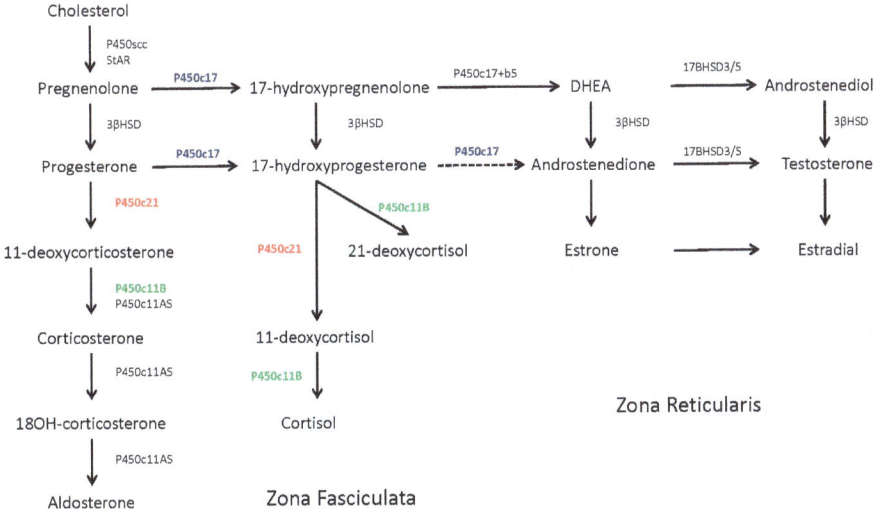

Figure 1. Adrenal steroidogenesis pathway. Biosynthetic pathway of mineralocorticoids (aldosterone), glucocorticoids (cortisol), and sex hormones (testosterone) within the adrenal. Partitioning for synthesis of key steroids occurring within each of the three zones (zonal glomerulosa, zona fasciculate, and zona reticularis) is provided in the shaded areas. Dashed lines with arrow heads, as compared to solid lines, denotes enzyme steps have limited affinity for conversion of the substrate to the product. DHEA = dehydroepiandrosterone, 3βHSD = 3β-hydroxysteroid dehydrogenase.

17OHP accumulates because human 17,20 lyase (P450c17) has limited to no capacity to convert it into androstenedione [8] (P450c17, in blue, Figure 1). The excess 17OHP is converted into androgens, specifically dihydroxytestosterone, via 'backdoor' pathways, or into an alternative product, 21-deoxycortisol, by 11β-hydroxylase (P450c11B) [9] (P450c11B, in green, Figure 1). Recent studies have noted the utility of 21-deoxycortisol, in addition to 17OHP, as a diagnostic marker for 21OHD [10]. 21-deoxycortisol is further converted into other 11-oxygentate androgens, which may also serve as useful biomarkers for disease identification and/or treatment management [11,12].

2.3. Genetics

21OHD is an autosomal recessive disorder caused by mutations in the *CYP21A2*. Interestingly, approximately 95% of the *CYP21A2* mutations are due to recombination events with its pseudogene (*CYP21P*) [13]. During mitosis, gene conversion with *CYP21P* introduces deleterious mutations into *CYP21A2*, while during meiosis, recombination events between the two genes cause deletions and creation of chimeric pseudogenes. More than 60 additional unique mutations in *CYP21A2* account for the remaining 5% of cases [13].

Adrenal P450 enzymes are controlled at the level of transcription and therefore the genotype-phenotype correlation is typically consistent. Deletions and nonsense mutations ablate enzyme activity and are most often associated with SW-CAH. Missense mutations typically yield 1–2% activity and are associated with SV-CAH. However, milder missense variants can produce 20–60% activity and be associated with NC-CAH [14]. In addition, patients may carry more than one mutation on either *CYP21A2* allele(s), leading to variances in severity within the three forms of CAH.

2.4. Diagnosis and Treatment

Infants with newborn screen results suggestive of 21OHD should be referred to and assessed by a pediatric endocrinologist. Elevated serum 17OHP levels can confirm 21OHD, and measurement of serum electrolytes and plasma renin activity identify newborns at risk of a salt-wasting crisis. A corticotropin stimulation test may be necessary when 17OHP levels are only mildly increased and diagnosis is unclear. Genotyping may assist with the interpretation of equivocal biochemical results and provide guidance for the genetic counseling of families [1].

Children with classic 21OHD require long-term glucocorticoid replacement treatment. The treatment goal is to suppress excess secretion of adrenal androgens using the lowest effective dose of glucocorticoid, typically hydroxycortisone, because glucocorticoid overtreatment is associated with growth suppression, weight gain and reduced bone mineral density. Infants with classic 21OHD are also treated with supplemental mineralocorticoids, typically fludrocortisone, coupled with sodium chloride replacement. Older children have reduced requirements for mineralocorticoid, although fludrocortisone may still be given as a glucocorticoid-sparing agent [1,9].

2.5. Newborn Screening

Newborn screening (NBS) for 21OHD was first initiated in Alaska in 1978 and became mandatory in all 50 states by 2009 [15]. The principal goal for screening is to facilitate the early detection of patients with severe 21OHD (SW-CAH), within the first week of life, to prevent the mortality and morbidity associated with salt-wasting crisis [1]. Historical publications demonstrate that screening readily detects the majority of patients with SW-CAH, while patients with SV-CAH are less reliably identified [7]. NC-CAH is not a target disease for NBS programs; however, there are reports of cases identified through screening [16].

17OHP is the primary marker used to identify newborns at risk for 21OHD. Initially, screening laboratories quantified 17OHP with a radioimmunoassay; however, this has since been replaced with a dissociation-enhanced lanthanide fluorescence immunoassay in automated systems (DELFIA). Typically, newborn screening laboratories set 17OHP cutoff values at low thresholds in attempts to detect all newborns with either form of classic 21OHD (100% screening sensitivity). However, this practice results in a large number of screened positive cases (cases in which 17OHP is elevated) of which very few are confirmed to have the disease (low positive predictive value (PPV)) [17]. 17OHP is elevated in both preterm and sick newborns, and typically males have higher 17OHP concentrations than females [7,18]. These factors have lead laboratories to adjust cutoff values based upon the baby's sex, birth weight and/or gestational age [19–24], yet in general, the positive predictive value remains low (on average less than 10%) for the first-tier immunoassay performed on specimens collected within the first two days of life [25]. Lastly, there are reports of missed cases of severe SW-CAH, because measured 17OHP concentrations were below set thresholds [26], suggesting that even lower cutoffs may be needed for the first-tier assay [27]. Of note, direct comparison of published laboratory screening algorithms using PPV can be challenging due to differences in unique protocols and definitions of screened positive cases. A summary of current testing algorithms and specimen collection practices, which have improved accuracy of the screen, is presented in Section 5.

Over the past 15 years, newborn screening programs have increasingly used second-tier biochemical testing, in addition to the first-tier immunoassay, to improve specificity. This practice of two-tier testing was endorsed in the 2018 Endocrine Society Clinical Practice Guidelines [1]. The second-tier assay, performed on the original specimen, quantifies 17OHP plus additional steroids, including cortisol, 21-deoxycortisol, and androstenedione, using liquid chromatography tandem mass spectrometry. Various combinations of individual steroid concentrations and ratios have been demonstrated to enhance screening specificity, decreasing false positive rates by as much as 90% [28,29]. In a recent prospective study, a reported PPV of 17% was achieved with a screening algorithm that included both first-tier immunoassay and second-tier steroid profiling [30]. Several laboratories have also shown increased specificity after implementing molecular analysis as a second-tier test; however,

3. Fetal Hypothalamic-Pituitary-Adrenal Axis and Adrenal Steroidogenesis

In this section, we outline normal fetal development and the initiation of independent adrenal steroidogenesis, highlighting how changes in maternal and placental signaling hormones effect production of fetal cortisol and other steroids, including 17OHP. This detailed analysis will set a context for later sections in which the reasons for both false positive and false negative screening results are explored.

3.1. Function of the HPA Axis

The hypothalamic-pituitary-adrenal (HPA) axis is the primary regulator of homeostasis within the body, managing resources during resting states, periods of high activity, and extreme stress. As summarized in the review by Howland et al., the stress stimulated cascade of hormone release begins with the production of corticotropin-releasing hormone (CRH) within neurons of the hypothalamus. Secreted CRH binds to receptors within the anterior pituitary and stimulates the release of adrenocorticotropic hormone (ACTH) [33]. ACTH then activates the steroidogenesis pathways in all zones within the adrenal cortex to maintain P450 expression and produce mineralocorticoids, glucocorticoids, and sex hormones. The newly synthesized glucocorticoid, cortisol, activates metabolism, and utilization of energy stores, regulates blood pressure, reduces inflammation, and enhances memory and attention. The stress response is terminated when excess circulating cortisol acts on glucocorticoid receptors in the hypothalamus and pituitary, inhibiting release of CRH and ACTH, respectively [33].

3.2. Adrenal Steroidogenesis

Unesterified cholesterol, derived from circulating low-density lipoprotein, is the precursor for adrenal steroidogenesis. The steroidogenic acute regulatory protein (StAR) assists in the transport of cholesterol from the cytosol to the inner mitochondria membrane to be converted into pregnenolone using the P450 side-chain cleavage (P450scc) enzyme. Pregnenolone then enters the smooth endoplasmic reticulum, where it is further converted to specific steroids, depending upon the compliment of other required enzymes [4]. The zona fasciculate of the adult adrenal contains abundant 17α-hydroxylase activity (P450c17), along with 3β-hydroxysteroid dehydrogenase (3βHSD), 21-hydroxylase (P450c21), and 11β-hydroxylase (P450c11B), which are all necessary for the production of cortisol from pregnenolone. The zona glomerulosa lacks the 17α-hydroxylase enzyme, committing pregnenolone to the exclusive production of aldosterone. In contrast, the zona reticularis in the adult adrenal contains 17α-hydroxylase and abundant cytochrome b5, which supports 17,20 lyase activity by the P450c17 protein. Of note, human 17,20 lyase activity favors production of dehydroepiandrosterone (DHEA), not androstenedione, which is rapidly used by other tissues for testosterone production [4,10]. The complete steroidogenic pathway with partitioning for each zone is shown in Figure 1.

3.3. Maternal, Placental, and Fetal Unit

During the prenatal period, the placenta acts at the interface between the maternal and fetal compartments, producing hormones that adjust maternal physiology to benefit mother and baby. Placental CRH, expressed by week 7 of gestation, is identical to maternal CRH, and functions to co-regulate stress hormone production during pregnancy. Specifically, placental CRH stimulates synthesis and release of maternal ACTH and downstream production of maternal cortisol from the adrenals. In a positive feedback loop, maternal cortisol then stimulates production of additional placental CRH (Figure 2) [33].

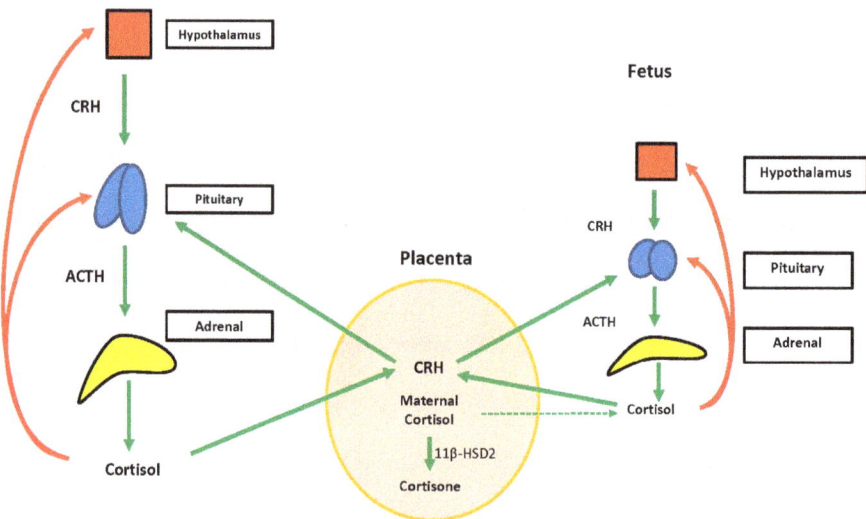

Figure 2. Maternal, placental, fetal unit. A representation of the hormone exchange between the maternal, fetal, and placental units. The maternal hypothalamic-pituitary-adrenal (HPA) axis stimulates cortisol production. Maternal cortisol is transferred to the placenta and converted into cortisone by 11β-HSD2, with only minimal exposure of the fetus to cortisol (dashed green line). Maternal cortisol also stimulates production of placental corticotropin-releasing hormone (CRH), which in turn activates synthesis and release of additional maternal adrenocorticotropic hormone (ACTH), creating a positive feedback loop (green arrows). Placental CRH also enters the fetal circulation and stimulates release of ACTH, which allows for production of fetal cortisol. Fetal cortisol stimulates additional placental CRH production creating a second positive feedback loop. Excess cortisol inhibits production of CRH and ACTH both within the maternal and fetal units (red arrows). Figure was modified from the Howland et al. (2017) reference [33].

During the prenatal period, the structures of the fetal HPA axis are undergoing tremendous growth, but the independent sequential release of fetal CRH, ACTH, and cortisol is not established until the third trimester [33]. The fetal stress response relies heavily upon the input of maternal and placental hormones. Placental CRH enters the fetal circulation and directly stimulates the fetal pituitary to release ACTH and the fetal adrenal to increase overall responsiveness to ACTH. This allows for production of systemic fetal cortisol as early as 24 weeks gestation. Fetal cortisol stimulates additional placental CRH production, similar to maternal cortisol, creating a second positive feedback loop (Figure 2) [33].

Exposure of the fetus to the exponential output of maternal cortisol is moderated by the placenta because excess maternal cortisol can otherwise inhibit fetal pituitary ACTH release. Specifically, the placental enzyme 11β-hydroxysteroid dehydrogenase 2 (11β-HSD2) oxidizes the biologically active maternal cortisol into its inactive form, cortisone [34], such that only a minimal amount of maternal cortisol will enter fetal circulation. However, by 34–35 weeks gestation, the activity of placental 11β-HSD2 decreases, allowing a surge of maternal cortisol into fetal compartments, which facilitates fetal organ maturation and enhances neurodevelopment prior to delivery [33,35] (Figure 3).

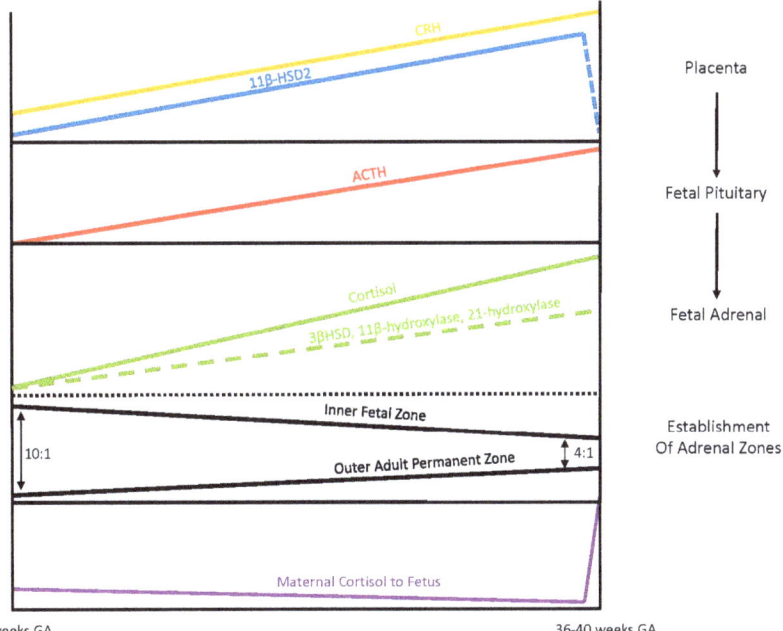

Figure 3. Dynamic changes of the fetal hypothalamic-pituitary-adrenal axis. During the third trimester, 24 to 36–40 weeks of gestation, the placenta increases production of corticotropin-releasing hormone (CRH). In response to placental CRH, production of adrenocorticotropic hormone (ACTH) by the fetal pituitary accelerates and stimulates the fetal adrenal to undergo steroidogenesis for cortisol production. Required enzymes for cortisol production within the adrenal, 3β- hydroxysteroid dehydrogenase (3βHSD), 21-hydroxylase (P450c21), 11β-hydroxylase, are activated. The establishment of the outer adult permanent zone of the adrenal also occurs during the third trimester. During the third trimester, activity of 11β-hydroxysteroid dehydrogenase 2 (11β-HSD2) within the placenta also increases and thereby exposure of the fetus to maternal cortisol remains low until the surge right before delivery. Figure was modified from the Howland et al. (2017) reference [33].

3.4. Fetal Adrenal Steroidogenesis

The fetal adrenal cortex is one of the most vascularized and active organs in early gestation, consisting of both an inner fetal zone and the outer adult or permanent zone [33]. In term infants, the ratio of the fetal zone to the adult zone is about 4 to 1, but the ratio is increased with lower gestational ages because the permanent zone matures later in response to the fetal pituitary hormone ACTH production [36]. The inner fetal zone originates in early development with the main function to produce DHEA, a precursor of estrogen, which is critically important for maternal adaption to pregnancy. For this reason, early fetal adrenals have low expression of 3β-HSD diverting all steroid precursors to DHEA [37,38]. However, from 24 weeks onward, fetal 3β-HSD activity in the permanent zone begins to increase, allowing independent synthesis of cortisol. By term, 75% of cortisol in fetal circulation is of fetal origin [33,39]. Taken together, these different stages of fetal adrenal development suggest that the abundance of steroidogenic precursors and products may differ between preterm and full-term newborns (Figure 3).

3.5. Preterm and Sick Infants

Multiple studies have demonstrated that basal cortisol concentrations in preterm and full-term newborns are comparable. Interestingly, the cortisol levels in both sick and healthy preterm newborns are also similar [40,41]. While cortisol levels would be anticipated to increase in preterm and sick newborns due to a stress response, this does not appear to be the case and it is possible that appropriate mechanisms to initiate a stress response are lacking. For cortisol synthesis to occur in response to stress, two actions are required. The fetal HPA axis must be intact to recognize stress and be capable of signal release of CRH by the hypothalamus and ACTH by the pituitary. Second, in response to ACTH stimulation, the adrenal enzymes must be present and functional to facilitate steroidogenesis. Several studies have evaluated both of these two required components to determine the underlying cause of reduced cortisol production in preterm newborns.

An early study investigated the function of the HPA axis in extremely low birth weight, stressed, premature infants. The infants were stimulated with either ovine CRH or ACTH and an appropriate ACTH or cortisol response was observed, respectively. As judged by the ability to respond to hormone stimulation, it was suggested that the pituitary and adrenal portions of the HPA axis appear to be intact as early as 26 weeks gestation [41]. A later study, evaluating preterm infants less than 32 weeks gestation age, confirmed the reports of previous study, demonstrating appropriate response to stressful stimuli by the elevation of ACTH [42]. These findings demonstrate a highly responsive HPA axis at early stages of the third trimester.

Other studies have directly evaluated adrenal steroidogenesis in full term newborns as compared to both premature healthy and sick newborns. The 17OHP, 11-deoxycortisol, and aldosterone concentrations were higher in sick preterm infants than in healthy preterm infants. Additionally, compared to full term newborns, preterm infants had significantly higher 17-hydroxypregnenolone, 17OHP, and DHEA sulfate concentrations. Cortisol and aldosterone values were not different between the sick and healthy preterm infants and were similar to concentrations measured in full term infants [43]. It was hypothesized from this data that adrenal enzyme activity in both healthy and sick preterm newborns is inadequate for production of cortisol. Further studies assessing enzyme function determined that 3β-HSD activity was not significantly reduced in extremely premature neonates, but activity of 11β-hydroxylase was markedly reduced [38]. Additional studies suggest that the activity of 21-hydroxylase is also decreased [36]. All authors concluded that very low birth weight premature infants are unable to mount a cortisol response due to deficiencies in multiple enzymes [44]. Accumulation of these steroid precursors, namely 17-hydroxypregnenolone and 17OHP, due to the decreased activity of successive enzymes, leads to a distribution of steroid concentrations that can actually mimic patterns observed in patients with 21-hydroxylase deficiency.

Throughout the third trimester, the adrenal continues to mature in response to pituitary activation and the permanent zone continues to delineate into three functional adult zones. This maturation process allows steroidogenic enzyme activities within the three zones to increase, resolving the back-up of steroid precursors, and allowing for independent cortisol synthesis at birth.

3.6. Effects of Glucocorticoid Treatment

Synthetic glucocorticoid administration is the standard of care for pregnant women at risk for premature delivery. This treatment promotes maturation of fetal organ systems to prepare the fetus for extra-uterine life however, excessive glucocorticoid exposure may have adverse effects on the fetus, including transient suppression of HPA activity [35,45]. Synthetic glucocorticoids pass through the placenta without being metabolized by 11β-HSD. Several studies showed that prenatal administration of synthetic glucocorticoids resulted in decreased cortisol production within the newborn for up to one week or longer after delivery [36,46]. Another study substantiated earlier reports by demonstrating that betamethasone blocked ACTH stimulation, leading to decreased expression of key steroid biosynthetic enzymes, P450scc, and 17-hydroxylase [45]. Depressed basal cortisol levels were also measured in newborns receiving dexamethasone or betamethasone treatment, and remained low for up to

7 days [40]. In general, however, the immediate and long-lasting impact of synthetic glucocorticoid administration on adrenal function in the newborn remains unclear and additional studies are needed to provide further clarification [32,42,46].

4. Review of False Positives and Negatives

In this next section we draw on what is known about the pathology of 21OHD, fetal HPA axis development, and adrenal steroidogenesis to explore reasons why both false positives and false negatives occur in newborn screening.

4.1. False Positives

It has been well documented by many laboratories that the first-tier immunoassay used to measure 17OHP as an indicator of 21OHD generates a large number of false positive cases, leading to a low positive predictive value for the first-tier screen (estimated to be less than 10%) [25]. From our assessment, false positives can be attributed to five potential sources, which are outlined below.

4.1.1. Physiological Changes in 17OHP Concentrations after Birth

The delivery of a newborn is a stressful event that causes elevations of multiple steroids, including 17OHP. 17OHP concentrations are higher in newborns right after birth and slowly decrease over a 24–48 h period. As demonstrated in an early report, median blood 17OHP concentrations in healthy term infants were greater than 100 nmol/L in cord blood, decreasing to 38 nmol/L by 12–18 h, and to 23 nmol/L by 24 h of life [47]. The implication of this data is that screening cutoffs should be adjusted to the time of collection [23]. If screening laboratories do not account for collection times, results from early sample collection (collected prior to 48 h of life) may be falsely identified as positive.

4.1.2. Immature Adrenal Function in Preterm Babies

Premature newborns produce large amounts of 17OHP due to adrenal enzyme immaturity. As outlined in the previous section, studies have demonstrated decreased activity of the 11β-hydroxylase enzyme in both healthy and sick premature infants and decreased 21-hydroxylase activity in babies born prior to 29 weeks [36,38]. Because adrenal steroidogenesis is not fully active in preterm babies, steroid precursors, including 17OHP, back up, leading to increased concentrations. All newborn screening programs should consider use of higher 17OHP cutoff values in premature babies, adjusting for gestational age and/or birthweight, to minimize false positives [21,24]. However, even with these stratifications of cutoff values, programs may still struggle with a low positive predictive value for the assay in premature newborns [7]. Section 5 below provides additional screening algorithm modifications to consider that can improve accuracy in preterm babies.

4.1.3. Stress Inducing Conditions of the Mother and Newborn

The fetal HPA axis responds to stress by driving an increase in ACTH and subsequent steroidogenesis, resulting in elevated concentrations of cortisol and steroid precursors, including 17OHP. Elevated 17OHP concentrations in newborns with respiratory distress syndrome has been documented in multiple studies [48]. Other fetal conditions associated with an elevated 17OHP concentration include hydrops fetalis, intraventricular hemorrhage, septicemia, congenital pneumonia, perinatal asphyxia, major abdominal surgical conditions, and severe congenital heart disease [49]. In mothers with pre-eclampsia, mean infant 17OHP levels were elevated and found to be associated with the presence of intrauterine growth restriction [50]. Therefore, fetal and maternal conditions can increased likelihood for a false positive screen. Physicians and laboratorians may wish to consider these complications when interpreting screening results.

4.1.4. Laboratory Methodologies

Performance of the 17OHP screening immunoassay is limited by antibody cross reactivity specifically with 17-hydroxypregnenolone sulfate, the major interfering compound [51]. This steroid is also found at higher concentrations in premature infants, as described in Section 3 above, contributing to the large number of false positive screens within premature babies. Immunoassay specificity can be improved with an initial extraction to remove cross-reacting steroid sulfates [52]. Measurement of 17OHP concentration by liquid chromatography-tandem mass spectrometry provides additional specificity, particularly among preterm infants [53]. Laboratories should consider use of a two-tier testing strategy to increase the accuracy of the screen.

4.1.5. Other Forms of CAH

It is important to mention that other forms of CAH cause elevations of 17OHP. Although significantly less common, accounting for fewer than 5% of all cases, CAH due to 11-hydroxylase deficiency, 3β-HSD deficiency, and P450 oxidoreductase deficiency can all present with elevated 17OHP levels [10]. Physicians and screening laboratories should be aware of the differential diagnosis for an elevated 17OHP.

4.2. False Negatives

In general, patients with severe 21OHD (SW-CAH) are readily detected by screening programs, while patients with simple-virilizing CAH, are less reliably identified. However, there are also reports of screening laboratories that have missed SW-CAH cases [26]. Below, we have identified five potential causes for low 17OHP values that can result in false negative cases.

4.2.1. Early Collection of Newborn Screening Specimen

17OHP values increase over time in untreated newborns affected with 21OHD [16,17,54]. Recent studies published by programs in the United States who routinely perform two newborn screens, have documented cases of both classic CAH (SW-CAH and SV-CAH) and NC-CAH identified on the second screen, due to late rising 17OHP concentrations [55–57]. Thus, screening accuracy for classic 21OHD, in particular for SV-CAH, may be relatively poor within the first 2 days of life when many screening laboratories collect specimens, increasing the risk of missed cases. Collection of a second screen could be considered as a means to improve screening accuracy. Additional details are provided in Section 5 below.

4.2.2. Immature Adrenal Function in Preterm Babies

During fetal development, the main function of the inner fetal zone of the adrenal is to produce dehydroepiandrosterone (DHEA). For this reason, early fetal adrenals have low expression of 3β-HSD, diverting all steroid precursors to production of DHEA [37,38]. However, within the third trimester, fetal 3β-HSD activity in the permanent zone begins to increase, enabling steroidogenesis and independent synthesis of cortisol [33,39]. The authors hypothesize that depending upon the stage of fetal adrenal development and the activity of the key enzyme 3β-HSD, the flux through the immature biosynthetic pathway of cortisol may not be adequate to elevate 17OHP concentrations in preterm newborns affected with 21OHD.

4.2.3. Increased Fetal Exposure to Maternal Cortisol

Maternal cortisol levels increase nearly 10-fold over the course of pregnancy and the placenta's role is to regulate fetal exposure to maternal cortisol, through the action of 11β-HSD. This regulation is incomplete and approximately 10% of maternal cortisol enters fetal circulation [33–35]. As described in Section 3, maternal cortisol suppresses both the production of fetal ACTH and its stimulation of steroidogenesis within the fetal adrenals. The authors hypothesize that excess maternal cortisol exposure may reduce flux through the fetal steroidogenic pathway, leading to decreased the amounts of 17OHP accumulation in patients with 21OHD, and a risk for missed cases by newborn screening.

4.2.4. Glucocorticoid Treatments

Conflicting evidence has been published on the suppressive effect of antenatal glucocorticoid treatments on pituitary adrenal function. The number of doses, the concentration of a single treatment, and the timing of when the last dose was administered can likely impact the magnitude of ACTH suppression resulting in decreased steroidogenic enzyme activities and subsequent reduction of cortisol synthesis. One study demonstrated that multiple courses of synthetic steroids in preterm infants decreased the 17OHP concentrations by ~30% in filter-paper blood [58]. Glucocorticoid treatments are a risk factor for adequate screening detection, due to the temporary reduction in 17OHP concentrations.

4.2.5. Mild Forms of 21-Hydroxylase Deficiency

As mentioned in previous sections, the activity of the 21-hydroxylase enzyme and the severity of the disease can be inferred from the 17OHP concentrations measured in untreated individuals. Patients with SW-CAH have the highest serum 17OHP levels, followed by patients with SV-CAH. Patients with NC-CAH have even smaller elevations, especially in the newborn period. Votava et al. estimated a false-negative rate of at least 33% in children with the moderate to mild forms of 21OHD [59]. Therefore, it should be well communicated to physicians that newborn screening is not adequate for identifying all patients with SV-CAH or NC-CAH.

5. Influence of Specimen Collection Times

In the previous section, we reviewed physiological factors, conditions of the newborn, and treatments that contribute to both false positive and false negative 21OHD screening results. Later specimen collection, after 48 h of life, can minimize many of the confounding factors that contribute to poor screening accuracy. However, any delay in specimen collection will also lead to a delay in diagnosis. Screening laboratories need to balance the accuracy of results with the urgency to detect newborns with 21OHD and other severe disorders on the newborn screening panel. Below is an abbreviated summary of specimen collection practices and outcomes reported by laboratories in the United States and other countries.

5.1. Screening in the United States

The timing of newborn screening specimen collection for programs in the United States has evolved over time in response to both changes in healthcare practices and federal recommendations. When screening began, blood specimens were typically collected between 48–96 h after birth, allowing time for key analytes to accumulate in response to dietary intake. Over time, collections began to occur earlier, even prior to 24 h of life, in response to early discharge practices within hospitals. To minimize the risk of a missed case, several states (currently 13 of the 50) incorporated a routine second screen, between 8–14 days of life, to provide a second opportunity to identify affected newborns. In 2015, the federal advisory committee on heritable disorders in newborns and children (ACHDNC) determined that, in order to facilitate timely diagnosis and treatment, the optimal time for specimen collection was between 24–48 h of life [60]. To our knowledge, all states have adopted this recommendation.

Early studies from Wisconsin and Texas reported identification of SW-CAH patients on the first screen at 1–2 days of life. However, milder forms of CAH (SV-CAH or NC-CAH) were either missed in Wisconsin, a one-screen state, or identified in Texas, a two-screen state, on the second screen [18,61]. Reports from Minnesota, Colorado, and the Northwest Regional Newborn Screening Program have also documented missed cases of both SW-CAH and SV-CAH on the first screen [26,56,57]. Colorado reported the sensitivity of their first screen as 71.8% for classic CAH (both SW-CAH and SV-CAH), with a false negative rate of 28.2% [56]. Similarly, the NWRSP stated that 25% of all confirmed cases of 21OHD were identified on the second screen. Of these infants identified on the second screen, 39% were classified as SW-CAH and 61% were classified as SV-CAH [57]. In 2015, a large multi-state comparison study found a similar detection rate for SW-CAH cases between one- and two-screen states; however, the detection rate for SV-CAH and NC-CAH was significantly higher in the two-screen states, with the majority being identified on the second screen. The study also reported missed cases of classic CAH in both one and two screen states, suggesting that delayed diagnoses may not be solely due to differences in collection practices [55].

In 2020, a nationwide US study comparing CAH screening protocols and outcomes, within a given year, was published [25]. The report included 17 states, of which 4 had a mandatory second screen. All but one of the 17 unique screening algorithms included cutoffs stratified by birthweight, and none of the states reported using a second-tier assay. The PPV ranged from 0.7% to 50% (mean 8.1%), with the two highest PPV found in two of the four states with mandatory second screen (50% and 20%). Taken together, this study, along with other historical reports, suggest that screening accuracy, defined as a high PPV, may be achieved through collection of a second specimen, along with an increased identification of milder forms of CAH (SV-CAH and NC-CAH); however, it may not eliminate the risk for missed, false negative, cases

Several states have implemented second-tier testing, using a steroid profile, for assessment of CAH (refer to Section 2.5). This practice, which is endorsed by the Endocrine Society Clinical Practice Guidelines, will also decrease false positive cases and improve the PPV. However, the majority of screening laboratories worldwide still only use a first-tier immunoassay. Additionally, second-tier testing will not address the risk for false negatives, due to the required reflex of an abnormal first-tier 17OHP concentration, as measured by the immunoassay.

5.2. Worldwide Screening

As of 2015, over 35 countries worldwide perform newborn screening for 21OHD with specimen collection typically occurring after 48 h of life, in contrast to the United States [3]. Below we review four recent publications from screening programs in Sweden, Israel, Brazil, and the Netherlands, and summarize how collection times have impacted screening sensitivity and the PPV of the assay. All of these programs screen for 21OHD using the 17OHP immunoassay, minimizing variability in outcomes due to differences in the screening tests.

A publication summarizing 26 years screening for 21OHD in Sweden reported 100% sensitivity for SW-CAH CAH and 80% sensitivity for SV-CAH [7]. All collections occurred after 48 h of life and cutoffs values were stratified by gestational age. The PPV of the screen was reported as 13.4% (25% for full term babies and 1.4% for preterm babies), which is significantly higher than that obtained by screening laboratories in the United States. Similarly, in a report from Israel, the screening sensitivity for classic CAH (SW-CAH and SV-CAH) was 95.4%, with an overall PPV of 16.5% [24]. Specimen collection occurred slightly earlier in this study, between 36–72 h of life, and cutoffs were stratified by both gestational age and birthweight.

Brazil published their screening algorithm in which the 17OHP cutoff levels were adjusted for the baby's birthweight and also age at specimen collection. Stratification of the population by two sampling time points, 48 to <72 h and ≥72 h, yielded a PPV of 5.6% and 14.1%, respectively, for the screen. No SW-CAH cases were missed. Collection prior to 48 h of life was strongly discouraged by the authors [62].

In 2019, the Dutch neonatal screening program published outcomes for 21OHD screening, with sample collection occurring between days 3–7 of life [6]. There were no missed SW cases and PPV was also high at 24.7%. However, several newborns presented unwell in a salt-wasting crisis prior to the physicians obtaining results from the screening laboratory. Due to the severity and early presentation of salt-wasting crisis in affected individuals, any delay in specimen collection may increase likelihood for detrimental outcomes.

All four of these studies address factors in normal physiology, such as the changing 17OHP concentrations after birth and the effects of prematurity on adrenal steroidogenesis that lead to decreased PPV of the first-tier screening assay. Accuracy of screening appears to be better when cutoff values are adjusted for the time of collection or by delaying specimen collection until after, at minimum, 48 h of life. However, all the authors' caution that delayed collection may lead to delayed diagnosis with the onset of symptoms prior to identification.

5.3. Screening in Premature Newborns

This review has detailed how adrenal immaturity, particularly in preterm newborns, contributes to reduced accuracy of 21OHD screening assays when samples are collected within the first few days of life. Many screening laboratories have observed this phenomenon and some have even proposed not screening preterm newborns because the positive predictive value of testing is too low; less than 0.4% PPV in a French report [63]. In addition, it could also be argued that preterm babies are already being monitored in a medical environment where there is minimal risk of missing a salt-wasting crisis.

Expert focus groups have recommended modified screening algorithms in premature babies to minimize the risk of both false negative and false positive screens. The Endocrine Society endorsed the Minnesota practice of rescreening premature, low birth weight infants (<1800 g) at 2 and 4 weeks of age [1,64]. Specifically, Minnesota demonstrated that timing of sample collection in premature babies played a more important role in reducing false positive results than implementation of second-tier testing [64]. Similarly, the Clinical Laboratory Standards Institute (CLSI) recommends that all preterm (<37 weeks gestation) and low birth weight (<2500 g) infants be screened on admission into the neonatal intensive care unit (NICU), and again at 48–72 h after birth, if the initial screen was performed at less than 24 h of life. A final screen is also recommended at 28 days of life [65]. Amongst the three groups, there is consensus that monitoring of 17OHP concentrations in premature newborns, 2–3 times within the first month of life, is needed to improve testing accuracy.

6. Conclusions

Early detection of 21OHD through newborn screening allows for treatment of most individuals prior to the onset of symptoms, preventing devastating outcomes from severe salt-wasting crises. The success of 21OHD screening can be assumed by the worldwide adoption of this disease onto screening panels. However, many programs report poor specificity with first-tier screening methods, leading to high false positive rates, and low positive predictive values. Likewise, limited sensitivity to detect all newborns with classic CAH is a significant concern.

In this review, we have summarized the pathology of 21OHD, along with the stages of fetal HPA axis development and functional adrenal steroidogenesis which contribute to reduced accuracy in screening assays. We highlight five factors that contribute to false positive cases and an additional five contributors to false negative cases. Lastly, we summarized how various approaches to specimen collection, used by screening laboratories worldwide, have impacted CAH screening performance. Adjustments for prematurity and timing of specimen collections post-delivery are major factors that must be considered in order to maximize the effectiveness of the screen.

It is hoped that this comprehensive review of key contributors to screening inaccuracies can provide insight for laboratorians, primary care physicians, and endocrinologists.

Funding: This research received no external funding.

Acknowledgments: The authors would like to acknowledge Lori Halverson for her contributions in editing and formatting of the manuscript for publication.

Conflicts of Interest: The authors declare no conflict of interest.

References

1. Speiser, P.W.; Arlt, W.; Auchus, R.J.; Baskin, L.S.; Conway, G.S.; Merke, D.P.; Meyer-Bahlburg, H.F.L.; Miller, W.L.; Murad, M.H.; Oberfield, S.E.; et al. Congenital Adrenal Hyperplasia Due to Steroid 21-Hydroxylase Deficiency: An Endocrine Society Clinical Practice Guideline. *J. Clin. Endocrinol. Metab.* **2018**, *103*, 4043–4088. [CrossRef]
2. Fox, D.A.; Ronsley, R.; Khowaja, A.R.; Haim, A.; Vallance, H.; Sinclair, G.; Amed, S. Clinical Impact and Cost Efficacy of Newborn Screening for Congenital Adrenal Hyperplasia. *J. Pediatr.* **2020**, *220*, 101–108. [CrossRef]
3. Therrell, B.L.; Padilla, C.D.; Loeber, J.G.; Kneisser, I.; Saadallah, A.; Borrajo, G.J.; Adams, J. Current Status of Newborn Screening Worldwide: 2015. *Semin. Perinatol.* **2015**, *39*, 171–187. [CrossRef]
4. Parsa, A.A.; New, M.I. Steroid 21-Hydroxylase Deficiency in Congenital Adrenal Hyperplasia. *J. Steroid Biochem. Mol. Biol.* **2017**, *165*, 2–11. [CrossRef] [PubMed]
5. Heather, N.L.; Seneviratne, S.N.; Webster, D.; Derraik, J.G.B.; Jefferies, C.; Carll, J.; Jiang, Y.; Cutfield, W.S.; Hofman, P.L. Newborn Screening for Congenital Adrenal Hyperplasia in New Zealand, 1994–2013. *J. Clin. Endocrinol. Metab.* **2015**, *100*, 1002–1008. [CrossRef] [PubMed]
6. Van Der Linde, A.A.A.; Schönbeck, Y.; van der Kamp, H.J.; Van Den Akker, E.L.T.; Van Albada, M.E.; Boelen, A.; Finken, M.J.J.; Hannema, S.E.; Hoorweg-Nijman, G.; Odink, R.J.; et al. Evaluation of the Dutch Neonatal Screening for Congenital Adrenal Hyperplasia. *Arch. Dis. Child.* **2019**, *104*, 653–657. [CrossRef] [PubMed]
7. Gidlöf, S.; Wedell, A.; Guthenberg, C.; Von Döbeln, U.; Nordenström, A. Nationwide Neonatal Screening for Congenital Adrenal Hyperplasia in Sweden. *JAMA Pediatr.* **2014**, *168*, 567. [CrossRef]
8. Conley, A.J.; Bird, I.M. The Role of Cytochrome P450 17α-Hydroxylase and 3β-Hydroxysteroid Dehydrogenase in the Integration of Gonadal and Adrenal Steroidogenesis via the Δ5 and Δ4 Pathways of Steroidogenesis in Mammals. *Biol. Reprod.* **1997**, *56*, 789–799. [CrossRef]
9. El-Maouche, D.; Arlt, W.; Merke, D.P. Congenital Adrenal Hyperplasia. *Lancet* **2017**, *390*, 2194–2210. [CrossRef]
10. Miller, W.L. Congenital Adrenal Hyperplasia: Time to Replace 17OHP with 21-Deoxycortisol. *Horm. Res. Paediatr.* **2019**, *91*, 416–420. [CrossRef]
11. White, P.C. Update on Diagnosis and Management of Congenital Adrenal Hyperplasia Due to 21-Hydroxylase Deficiency. *Curr. Opin. Endocrinol. Diabetes Obes.* **2018**, *25*, 178–184. [CrossRef] [PubMed]
12. Turcu, A.F.; Mallappa, A.; Elman, M.S.; Avila, N.A.; Marko, J.; Rao, H.; Tsodikov, A.; Auchus, R.J.; Merke, D.P. 11-Oxygenated Androgens Are Biomarkers of Adrenal Volume and Testicular Adrenal Rest Tumors in 21-Hydroxylase Deficiency. *J. Clin. Endocrinol. Metab.* **2017**, *102*, 2701–2710. [CrossRef] [PubMed]
13. Speiser, P.W.; White, P.C. Congenital Adrenal Hyperplasia. *N. Engl. J. Med.* **2003**, *349*, 776–788. [CrossRef] [PubMed]
14. Falhammar, H.; Wedell, A.; Nordenström, A. Biochemical and Genetic Diagnosis of 21-Hydroxylase Deficiency. *Endocrine* **2015**, *50*, 306–314. [CrossRef]
15. Pang, S.; Spence, D.A.; New, M.I. Newborn screening for congenital adrenal hyperplasia with special reference to screening in Alaska. *Ann. N. Y. Acad. Sci.* **1985**, *458*, 90–102. [CrossRef]
16. Therrell, B.L.; Berenbaum, S.A.; Manter-Kapanke, V.; Simmank, J.; Korman, K.; Prentice, L.; Gonzalez, J.; Gunn, S. Results of Screening 1.9 Million Texas Newborns for 21-Hydroxylase-Deficient Congenital Adrenal Hyperplasia. *Pediatrics* **1998**, *101*, 583–590. [CrossRef]
17. White, P.C. Optimizing Newborn Screening for Congenital Adrenal Hyperplasia. *J. Pediatr.* **2013**, *163*, 10–12. [CrossRef]
18. Varness, T.S.; Allen, D.B.; Hoffman, G.L. Newborn Screening for Congenital Adrenal Hyperplasia Has Reduced Sensitivity in Girls. *J. Pediatr.* **2005**, *147*, 493–498. [CrossRef]
19. Sarafoglou, K.; Banks, K.; Gavigio, A.; McCann, M.; Thomas, W. Comparison of One-Tier and Two-Tier Newborn Screening Metrics for Congenital Adrenal Hyperplasia. *Pediatrics* **2012**, *130*, e1261–e1268. [CrossRef]
20. Allen, D.B.; Hoffman, G.L.; Fitzpatrick, P.; Laessig, R.; Maby, S.; Slyper, A. Improved Precision of Newborn Screening for Congenital Adrenal Hyperplasia Using Weight-Adjusted Criteria for 17-Hydroxyprogesterone Levels. *J. Pediatr.* **1997**, *130*, 128–133. [CrossRef]

21. Olgemöller, B.; Roscher, A.A.; Liebl, B.; Fingerhut, R. Screening for Congenital Adrenal Hyperplasia: Adjustment of 17-Hydroxyprogesterone Cut-Off Values to Both Age and Birth Weight Markedly Improves the Predictive Value. *J. Clin. Endocrinol. Metab.* **2003**, *88*, 5790–5794. [CrossRef] [PubMed]
22. Van Der Kamp, H.J.; Oudshoorn, C.G.M.; Elvers, B.H.; Baarle, M.V.; Otten, B.J.; Wit, J.M.; Verkerk, P.H. Cutoff Levels of 17-α-Hydroxyprogesterone in Neonatal Screening for Congenital Adrenal Hyperplasia Should Be Based on Gestational Age Rather Than on Birth Weight. *J. Clin. Endocrinol. Metab.* **2005**, *90*, 3904–3907. [CrossRef] [PubMed]
23. Jiang, X.; Tang, F.; Feng, Y.; Li, B.; Jia, X.; Tang, C.; Liu, S.; Juang, Y. The adjustment of 17-hydroxyprogesterone cut-off values for congenital adrenal hyperplasia neonatal screening by GSP according to gestational age and age at sampling. *J. Pediatr. Endocrinol. Metab.* **2019**, *32*, 1253–1258. [CrossRef]
24. Pode-Shakked, N.; Blau, A.; Pode-Shakked, B.; Tiosano, D.; Weintrob, N.; Eyal, O.; Zung, A.; Levy-Khademi, F.; Tenenbaum-Rakover, Y.; Zangen, D.; et al. Combined Gestational Age- and Birth Weight–Adjusted Cutoffs for Newborn Screening of Congenital Adrenal Hyperplasia. *J. Clin. Endocrinol. Metab.* **2019**, *104*, 3172–3180. [CrossRef] [PubMed]
25. Speiser, P.W.; Chawla, R.; Chen, M.; Diaz-Thomas, A.; Finlayson, C.; Rutter, M.M.; Sandberg, D.E.; Shimy, K.; Talib, R.; Cerise, J.; et al. Disorders/Differences of Sex Development-Translational Research Network (DSD-TRN) Newborn screening protocols and positive predictive value for congenital adrenal hyperplasia vary across the United States. *Int. J. Neonatal Screen.* **2020**, *6*, 37. [CrossRef]
26. Sarafoglou, K.; Banks, K.; Kyllo, J.; Pittock, S.; Thomas, W. Cases of Congenital Adrenal Hyperplasia Missed by Newborn Screening in Minnesota. *JAMA* **2012**, *307*, 2371–2374. [CrossRef]
27. Lasarev, M.R.; Bialk, E.R.; Allen, D.B.; Held, P.K. Application of Principal Component Analysis to Newborn Screening for Congenital Adrenal Hyperplasia. *J. Clin. Endocrinol. Metab.* **2020**, *105*, 1–11. [CrossRef]
28. Lacey, J.M.; Minutti, C.Z.; Magera, M.J.; Tauscher, A.L.; Casetta, B.; Mccann, M.; Lymp, J.; Hahn, S.H.; Rinaldo, P.; Matern, D. Improved Specificity of Newborn Screening for Congenital Adrenal Hyperplasia by Second-Tier Steroid Profiling Using Tandem Mass Spectrometry. *Clin. Chem.* **2004**, *50*, 621–625. [CrossRef]
29. Schwarz, E.; Liu, A.; Randall, H.; Haslip, C.; Keune, F.; Murray, M.; Longo, N.; Pasquali, M. Use of Steroid Profiling by UPLC-MS/MS as a Second Tier Test in Newborn Screening for Congenital Adrenal Hyperplasia: The Utah Experience. *Pediatr. Res.* **2009**, *66*, 230–235. [CrossRef]
30. Bialk, E.; Lasarev, M.R.; Held, P.K. Wisconsin's Screening Algorithm for the Identification of Newborns with Congenital Adrenal Hyperplasia. *Int. J. Neonatal Screen.* **2019**, *5*, 33. [CrossRef]
31. Kopacek, C.; Prado, M.J.; Silva, C.M.D.; De Castro, S.M.; Beltrão, L.A.; Vargas, P.R.; Grandi, T.; Rossetti, M.L.; Spritzer, P.M. Clinical and Molecular Profile of Newborns with Confirmed or Suspicious Congenital Adrenal Hyperplasia Detected after a Public Screening Program Implementation. *J. Pediatr.* **2019**, *95*, 282–290. [CrossRef] [PubMed]
32. Nordenstrom, A.; Wedell, A.; Hagenfeldt, L.; Marcus, C.; Larsson, A. Neonatal Screening for Congenital Adrenal Hyperplasia: 17-Hydroxyprogesterone Levels and CYP21 Genotypes in Preterm Infants. *Pediatrics* **2001**, *108*, E68. [CrossRef] [PubMed]
33. Howland, M.A.; Sandman, C.A.; Glynn, L.M. Developmental Origins of the Human Hypothalamic-Pituitary-Adrenal Axis. *Expert Rev. Endocrinol. Metab.* **2017**, *12*, 321–339. [CrossRef] [PubMed]
34. Liu, Q.; Jin, S.; Sun, X.; Sheng, X.; Mao, Z.; Jiang, Y.; Liu, H.; Hu, C.; Xia, W.; Li, Y.; et al. Maternal Blood Pressure, Cord Glucocorticoids, and Child Neurodevelopment at 2 Years of Age: A Birth Cohort Study. *Am. J. Hypertens.* **2019**, *32*, 524–530. [CrossRef]
35. Zhu, P.; Wang, W.; Zuo, R.; Sun, K. Mechanisms for Establishment of the Placental Glucocorticoid Barrier, a Guard for Life. *Cell. Mol. Life Sci.* **2019**, *76*, 13–26. [CrossRef]
36. Nomura, S. Immature Adrenal Steroidogenesis in Preterm Infants. *Early Hum. Dev.* **1997**, *49*, 225–233. [CrossRef]
37. Wang, W.; Chen, Z.-J.; Myatt, L.; Sun, K. 11β-HSD1 in Human Fetal Membranes as a Potential Therapeutic Target for Preterm Birth. *Endocr. Rev.* **2018**, *39*, 241–260. [CrossRef]
38. Hingre, R.V.; Gross, S.J.; Hingre, K.S.; Mayes, D.M.; Richman, R.A. Adrenal Steroidogenesis in Very Low Birth Weight Preterm Infants. *J. Clin. Endocrinol. Metab.* **1994**, *78*, 266–270. [CrossRef]

39. Kosicka, K.; Siemiątkowska, A.; Szpera-Goździewicz, A.; Krzyścin, M.; Bręborowicz, G.H.; Główka, F.K. Increased Cortisol Metabolism in Women with Pregnancy-Related Hypertension. *Endocrine* **2018**, *61*, 125–133. [CrossRef]
40. Kari, M.A.; Raivio, K.O.; Stenman, U.H.; Voutilainen, R. Serum Cortisol, Dehydroepiandrosterone Sulfate, and Steroid-Binding Globulins in Preterm Neonates: Effect of Gestational Age and Dexamethasone Therapy. *Pediatr. Res.* **1996**, *40*, 319–324. [CrossRef] [PubMed]
41. Hanna, C.E.; Keith, L.D.; Colasurdo, M.A.; Buffkin, D.C.; Laird, M.R.; Mandel, S.H.; Cook, D.M.; Lafranchi, S.H.; Reynolds, J.W. Hypothalamic Pituitary Adrenal Function in the Extremely Low Birth Weight Infant. *J. Clin. Endocrinol. Metab.* **1993**, *76*, 384–387. [CrossRef] [PubMed]
42. Ng, P.C.; Wong, G.W.K.; Lam, C.W.K.; Lee, C.H.; Wong, M.Y.; Fok, T.F.; Wong, W.; Chan, D.C.F. Pituitary-Adrenal Response in Preterm Very Low Birth Weight Infants after Treatment with Antenatal Corticosteroids. *J. Clin. Endocrinol. Metab.* **1997**, *82*, 3548–3552. [CrossRef] [PubMed]
43. Lee, M.M.; Rajagopalan, L.; Berg, G.J.; Moshang, T. Serum Adrenal Steroid Concentrations in Premature Infants. *J. Clin. Endocrinol. Metab.* **1989**, *69*, 1133–1136. [CrossRef] [PubMed]
44. Korte, C.; Styne, D.; Merritt, T.; Mayes, D.; Wertz, A.; Helbock, H.J. Adrenocortical Function in the Very Low Birth Weight Infant: Improved Testing Sensitivity and Association with Neonatal Outcome. *J. Pediatr.* **1996**, *128*, 257–263. [CrossRef]
45. Kessel, J.M.; Cale, J.M.; Verbrick, E.; Parker, C.R.; Carlton, D.P.; Bird, I.M. Antenatal Betamethasone Depresses Maternal and Fetal Aldosterone Levels. *Reprod. Sci.* **2008**, *16*, 94–104. [CrossRef] [PubMed]
46. Ballard, P.L.; Gluckman, P.D.; Liggins, G.C.; Kaplan, S.L.; Grumbach, M.M. Steroid and Growth Hormone Levels in Premature Infants After Prenatal Betamethasone Therapy to Prevent Respiratory Distress Syndrome. *Pediatr. Res.* **1980**, *14*, 122–127. [CrossRef]
47. Gruñeiro De Papendieck, L.; Prieto, L.; Chiesa, A.; Bengolea, S.; Bergadá, C. Congenital Adrenal Hyperplasia and Early Newborn Screening: 17α-Hydroxyprogesterone (17α-OHP) during the First Days of Life. *J. Med. Screen.* **1998**, *5*, 24–26. [CrossRef]
48. Ryckman, K.K.; Cook, D.E.; Berberich, S.L.; Shchelochkov, O.A.; Berends, S.K.; Busch, T.; Dagle, J.M.; Murray, J.C. Replication of Clinical Associations with 17-Hydroxyprogesterone in Preterm Newborns. *J. Pediatr. Endocrinol. Metab.* **2012**, *25*, 301–305. [CrossRef]
49. Murphy, J.F.; Joyce, B.G.; Dyas, J.; Hughes, I.A. Plasma 17-Hydroxyprogesterone Concentrations in Ill Newborn Infants. *Arch. Dis. Child.* **1983**, *58*, 532–534. [CrossRef]
50. Ersch, J.; Beinder, E.; Stallmach, T.; Bucher, H.U.; Torresani, T. 17-Hydroxyprogesterone in Premature Infants as a Marker of Intrauterine Stress. *J. Perinat. Med.* **2008**, *36*, 157–160. [CrossRef]
51. Wong, T.; Shackleton, C.H.; Covey, T.R.; Ellis, G. Identification of the Steroids in Neonatal Plasma That Interfere with 17 Alpha-Hydroxyprogesterone Radioimmunoassays. *Clin. Chem.* **1992**, *38*, 1830–1837. [CrossRef] [PubMed]
52. Fingerhut, R. False Positive Rate in Newborn Screening for Congenital Adrenal Hyperplasia (CAH)–Ether Extraction Reveals Two Distinct Reasons for Elevated 17α-Hydroxyprogesterone (17-OHP) Values. *Steroids* **2009**, *74*, 662–665. [CrossRef] [PubMed]
53. De Hora, M.R.; Heather, N.L.; Patel, T.; Bresnahan, L.G.; Webster, D.; Hofman, P.L. Measurement of 17-Hydroxyprogesterone by LCMSMS Improves Newborn Screening for CAH Due to 21-Hydroxylase Deficiency in New Zealand. *Int. J. Neonatal Screen.* **2020**, *6*, 6. [CrossRef]
54. Nordenstrom, A.; Thilen, A.; Hagenfeldt, L.; Larsson, A.; Wedell, A. Genotyping is a valuable diagnostic complement to neonatal screening for congenital adrenal hyperplasia due to steroid 21-hydroxylase deficiency. *J. Clin. Endocrinol. Metab.* **1999**, *84*, 1505–1509. [CrossRef] [PubMed]
55. Held, P.K.; Shapira, S.K.; Hinton, C.F.; Jones, E.; Hannon, W.H.; Ojodu, J. Congenital Adrenal Hyperplasia Cases Identified by Newborn Screening in One- and Two-Screen States. *Mol. Genet. Metab.* **2015**, *116*, 133–138. [CrossRef] [PubMed]
56. Chan, C.L.; Mcfann, K.; Taylor, L.; Wright, D.; Zeitler, P.S.; Barker, J.M. Congenital Adrenal Hyperplasia and the Second Newborn Screen. *J. Pediatr.* **2013**, *163*, 109–113. [CrossRef]
57. Eshragh, N.; Van Doan, L.; Connelly, K.J.; Denniston, S.; Willis, S.; LaFranchi, S.H. Oucome of newborn screening for congenital adrenal hyperplasia at two time points. *Horm. Res. Pediatr.* **2020**, *93*, 128–136. [CrossRef]

58. Gatelais, F.; Berthelot, J.; Beringue, F.; Descamps, P.; Bonneau, D.; Limal, J.-M.; Coutant, R. Effect of Single and Multiple Courses of Prenatal Corticosteroids on 17-Hydroxyprogesterone Levels: Implication for Neonatal Screening of Congenital Adrenal Hyperplasia. *Pediatr. Res.* **2004**, *56*, 701–705. [CrossRef]
59. Votava, F.; Dóra, T.; József, K.; Dorothea, M.; Baumgartner-Parzer, S.M.; János, S.; Zuzana, P.; Battelino, T.; Lebl, J.; Frisch, H.; et al. Estimation of the False-Negative Rate in Newborn Screening for Congenital Adrenal Hyperplasia. *Eur. J. Endocrinol.* **2005**, *152*, 869–874. [CrossRef]
60. Newborn Screening Timeliness Goals. Official Website of the U.S. Health Resources & Services Administration. Available online: https://www.hrsa.gov/advisory-committees/heritable-disorders/newborn-screening-timeliness.html (accessed on 23 April 2020).
61. Brosnan, C.; Brosnan, P.; Therrell, B.L.; Slater, C.H.; Swint, J.M.; Annegers, J.F.; Riley, W.J. A Comparative Cost Analysis of Newborn Screening for Classic Congenital Adrenal Hyperplasia in Texas. *Public Health Rep.* **1998**, *113*, 170–178.
62. Hayashi, G.Y.; Carvalho, D.F.; Miranda, M.C.D.; Faure, C.; Vallejos, C.; Brito, V.N.; Rodrigues, A.D.S.; Madureira, G.; Mendonca, B.B.; Bachega, T.A. Neonatal 17-Hydroxyprogesterone Levels Adjusted According to Age at Sample Collection and Birthweight Improve the Efficacy of Congenital Adrenal Hyperplasia Newborn Screening. *Clin. Endocrinol.* **2017**, *86*, 480–487. [CrossRef] [PubMed]
63. Coulm, B. Efficiency of Neonatal Screening for Congenital Adrenal Hyperplasia Due to 21-Hydroxylase Deficiency in Children Born in Mainland France between 1996 and 2003. *Arch. Pediatr. Adolesc. Med.* **2012**, *166*, 113. [CrossRef] [PubMed]
64. Sarafoglou, K.; Gaviglio, A.; Hietala, A.; Frogner, G.; Banks, K.; Mccann, M.; Thomas, W. Comparison of Newborn Screening Protocols for Congenital Adrenal Hyperplasia in Preterm Infants. *J. Pediatr.* **2014**, *164*, 1136–1140. [CrossRef] [PubMed]
65. *NBS03 Newborn Screening for Preterm, Low Birth Weight, and Sick Newborns*, 2nd ed.; Clinical and Laboratory Standards Institute (CLSI): Wayne, PA, USA, 2019; Volume 39, pp. 11–29.

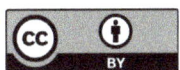

© 2020 by the authors. Licensee MDPI, Basel, Switzerland. This article is an open access article distributed under the terms and conditions of the Creative Commons Attribution (CC BY) license (http://creativecommons.org/licenses/by/4.0/).

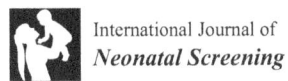

International Journal of
Neonatal Screening

Article

We All Have a Role to Play: Redressing Inequities for Children Living with CAH and Other Chronic Health Conditions of Childhood in Resource-Poor Settings

Kate Armstrong [1,2,*], Alain Benedict Yap [3], Sioksoan Chan-Cua [4], Maria E. Craig [5,6], Catherine Cole [1], Vu Chi Dung [7], Joseph Hansen [1], Mohsina Ibrahim [8], Hassana Nadeem [8], Aman Pulungan [9], Jamal Raza [8], Agustini Utari [10] and Paul Ward [2]

1. CLAN (Caring & Living As Neighbours), Denistone 2114, Australia; cath@clanchildhealth.org (C.C.); joehansen223@gmail.com (J.H.)
2. College of Medicine & Public Health, Flinders University, Adelaide 5042, Australia; paul.ward@flinders.edu.au
3. CAHSAPI (Congenital Adrenal Hyperplasia Support Group of the Philippines), Manila 1000, Philippines; alain@friarminor.com
4. Department of Pediatrics, Philippines General Hospital, Manila 1000, Philippines; sioksoan@gmail.com
5. Institute of Endocrinology and Diabetes, The Children's Hospital at Westmead/Discipline of Child and Adolescent Health, University of Sydney, Camperdown 2006, Australia; m.craig@unsw.edu.au
6. School of Women's and Children's Health, UNSW Medicine, Kensington 2052, Australia
7. Department of Pediatric Endocrinology and Metabolism, National Children's Hospital, Hanoi 100000, Vietnam; dungvu@nch.org.vn
8. National Institute of Child Health (NICH), Karachi 75510, Pakistan; mohsinaibrahim@yahoo.com (M.I.); drhassana70@yahoo.com (H.N.); drjamalraza@gmail.com (J.R.)
9. Department of Child Health University of Indonesia, Dr. Cipto Mangunkusumo Hospital, Jakarta 10430, Indonesia; amanpulungan@mac.com
10. Department of Pediatrics, Faculty of Medicine, Diponegoro University, Semarang 50275, Indonesia; agustiniutari@gmail.com
* Correspondence: kate@clanchildhealth.org

Received: 1 September 2020; Accepted: 21 September 2020; Published: 25 September 2020

Abstract: CLAN (Caring and Living as Neighbours) is an Australian-based non-governmental organisation (NGO) committed to equity for children living with chronic health conditions in resource-poor settings. Since 2004, CLAN has collaborated with a broad range of partners across the Asia Pacific region to improve quality of life for children living with congenital adrenal hyperplasia (CAH). This exploratory case study uses the Knowledge to Action (KTA) framework to analyse CLAN's activities for children living with CAH in the Asia Pacific. The seven stages of the KTA action cycle inform a systematic examination of comprehensive, collaborative, sustained actions to address a complex health challenge. The KTA framework demonstrates the "how" of CLAN's approach to knowledge creation and exchange, and the centrality of community development to multisectoral collaborative action across a range of conditions, cultures and countries to redressing child health inequities. This includes a commitment to: affordable access to essential medicines and equipment; education, research and advocacy; optimisation of medical management; encouragement of family support groups; efforts to reduce financial burdens; and ethical, transparent program management as critical components of success. Improvements in quality of life and health outcomes are achievable for children living with CAH and other chronic health conditions in resource-poor settings. CLAN's strategic framework for action offers a model for those committed to #LeaveNoChildBehind.

Keywords: congenital adrenal hyperplasia; inequity; community development; human rights; child; parents; community; chronic; non-communicable diseases; poverty

1. Introduction

Congenital adrenal hyperplasia (CAH) is a spectrum of autosomal recessive disorders of adrenal steroidogenesis, caused by an enzyme deficiency in the adrenal cortex (21-hydroxylase in approximately 95% of cases [1]). Reduced activity or absence of 21-hydroxlase impairs cortisol and aldosterone production, and diverts hormone biosynthesis precursors to excess androgen production. Whilst CAH is unquestionably a complex health condition to manage, internationally recognized clinical guidelines now provide evidence-based recommendations regarding the appropriate management of CAH to support affected individuals so they might enjoy the highest quality of life possible [1–3].

Despite this depth of knowledge—and the many educational materials, tools and other resources available to facilitate positive health outcomes—for some people living in low- and middle-income countries around the world in 2020 it could be argued that not much has changed since DeCrecchio's first description of CAH and the life and tragic premature death of Giuseppe Marzo back in 1865 [4]. In low-income countries where there is no newborn screening (NBS) for CAH [5], low prevalence, high mortality and unequal gender distribution (with male infants dying of undiagnosed salt-wasting crises) are more likely rapid quantitative indicators of inequities of access than they are of low incidence [6], with many of the world's children failing to benefit from the diagnostic and therapeutic solutions for CAH that have been evolving since the 1950s. Glucocorticoid (hydrocortisone, prednisone and dexamethasone) and mineralocorticoid (fludrocortisone) replacement therapies have proven safe and effective in the maintenance and emergency management of CAH for over 60 years, and NBS promotes timely diagnosis, yet neither are routinely nor affordably available globally at the present time. Indeed, inequities are not always exclusive to low- and middle-income countries: despite the clear advantages of NBS for CAH, some high-income countries (such as Australia) have still not implemented universal nationwide NBS programs, and the resultant preventable morbidity and mortality are increasingly difficult to justify [7–10].

In 1999, the lived experience of almost losing a three-week-old infant to an adrenal crisis caused by undiagnosed CAH led one Australian (author Kate Armstrong) to appreciate first-hand the dichotomous juxtaposition of the potential for extreme and preventable trauma associated with CAH, against the relative ease of achieving an excellent quality of life once a diagnosis was made and access to affordable, quality healthcare made available. In 2004, this newfound appreciation of the potential for CAH to impact differentially on peoples' lives was further enhanced by a growing awareness of the experiences of children and families living with CAH in Vietnam. Articles in Australian [11] and American [12] CAH support group newsletters spoke of widespread mortality and morbidity, financial devastation, social isolation and stigma associated with CAH in Vietnam, at a time when young people living in neighbouring countries such as Australia and New Zealand were celebrating personal, educational and vocational achievements in lives relatively unscathed by the same health condition. These reports raised important questions. What were the barriers and challenges faced by families in Vietnam, and what actions could be taken to redress the inequities? What might it take for every child living with CAH in Vietnam to enjoy a quality of life on par with that of children in Australia and other high-income countries around the world?

What Is Caring and Living as Neighbours (CLAN)?

Founded in 2004 in response to a growing awareness of adverse outcomes for children living with CAH in Vietnam, CLAN (Caring and Living as Neighbours) [13] is an Australian non-governmental organisation (NGO) committed to a rights-based approach to optimizing quality of life for children and young people living with CAH and other chronic health conditions in resource-poor settings.

A published survey of 53 families of children living with CAH in Vietnam in 2005 [14] led to the development of CLAN's rights-based, strategic framework for action (Figure 1) which seeks to focus multisectoral collaborative efforts on five pillars considered essential to achieving the highest quality of life possible for communities of children living with chronic health conditions:

1. Affordable access to essential medicines and equipment;
2. Education, research and advocacy;
3. Optimisation of medical management (with a focus on primary, secondary and tertiary prevention);
4. Encouragement of family support groups; and
5. Reducing financial burdens and promoting financial independence.

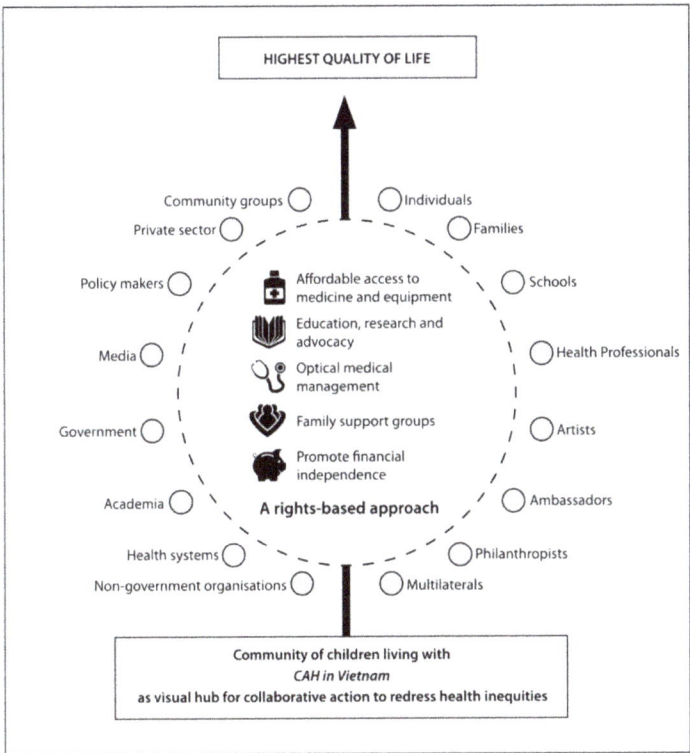

Figure 1. The Caring and Living as Neighbours (CLAN) Strategic Framework for Action (as developed to facilitate change for children living with congenital adrenal hyperplasia (CAH) in Vietnam).

CLAN's framework maintains communities of children living with specific chronic health conditions as the visual hub of multisectoral action, and advocates for community development and patient-and family-centred care. Refined over more than 15 years, and since translated to a broad range of other chronic conditions of childhood (including type 1 diabetes, osteogenesis imperfecta (OI), nephrotic syndrome, rheumatic heart disease and epilepsy), and applied across a number of cultures, communities and countries (including Indonesia, the Philippines, Pakistan, India, Kenya, Uganda and Fiji), CLAN's Strategic Framework for Action has proven a useful guide for engaging with new partners who are seeking to redress inequities for children with special health needs [15–17].

From a sustainability and scalability perspective, CLAN's goal is to share the "how" of implementing our strategic framework and "five pillars" so that others seeking to redress inequities associated with CAH and other chronic conditions of childhood can do so independently of CLAN. The authors acknowledge CAH as a complex health condition, for which comprehensive biomedical knowledge already exists regarding optimal lifelong management. The objective of this paper, therefore, is not to duplicate existing documented clinical and biomedical knowledge on CAH, but rather to describe the novel community development, multi-sectoral collaborative approach CLAN and our many partners and stakeholders have taken with regards CAH (and, later, other conditions) in Vietnam (and, later, other countries), to provide a model based on the knowledge, tools and products that have been developed over time that might be applicable to drive advocacy and action for CAH and other chronic conditions in other countries.

2. Materials and Methods

The underlying ontology, epistemology and methodology of this paper is explicitly acknowledged for full transparency.

The ontology of the first author of this paper (Kate Armstrong) is informed by personal circumstance (as the mother of a young person living with CAH in Australia); professional training (as a medical doctor and public health physician); and lived experience (as the founder and president of CLAN). The co-authors bring clinical and bio-medical expertise from Australia (Maria E Craig), Vietnam (Vu Chi Dung), the Philippines (Sioksoan Chan-Cua), Indonesia (Aman Pulungan, Agustini Utari) and Pakistan (Jamal Raza, Mohsina Ibrahim, Hassana Nadeem); as well as CAH Community (Joseph Hansen and Alain Benedict Yap), organisational (Catherine Cole), public health and sociological insights (Paul Ward). The positionality [18,19] of each co-author differs necessarily: as CAH community insiders and outsiders, medical and public health insiders, CLAN insiders, cultural insiders and outsiders, each brings unique power, knowledge and expertise to this analysis, and we acknowledge the many others who have contributed equally generously to collective efforts for CAH communities in the Asia Pacific region to date (please see Acknowledgements section of this paper).

The epistemological paradigm of critical realism [20] has informed the work of CLAN, and the organisation's underlying optimism that "change is possible" providing we continue to strive for deeper levels of explanation and understanding. The lived experiences of children and families living with chronic health conditions in resource poor settings are manifestations of underlying causal structures and mechanisms that, once understood and addressed, can be influenced and changed for the better [21,22]. Prioritising the voices of people living with chronic conditions (or the parents of children where their voices cannot yet be shared) reflects CLAN's commitment to valuing felt needs and patient and family-centred approaches [23], and prioritisation of participatory action research (PAR) when implementing CLAN's framework [24], and aligns with emerging calls to privilege the voices of people living with chronic conditions within the broader non-communicable disease (NCD) discourse [25].

The authors accept the imperfect nature of all information and knowledge presented, sharing it as a genuine attempt to communicate as objectively as possible a brief insight into the complex series of events, outcomes and impact observed over many years, across a number of countries and health conditions of childhood. A commitment to continuous quality improvement (CQI), reflection, strategic planning, monitoring and evaluation has informed CLAN's work since 2004, and this paper has been written in response to a request from the editors of the International Journal of Newborn Screening (IJNS) to document the work of CLAN in relation to CAH. As such, this paper does not seek to evaluate CLAN's work comprehensively and objectively (almost impossible given the authors' insider positionality), but rather describe and explain it.

The methodology of this research paper is that of an exploratory case study. This particular case study research design is often used to answer questions that ask the "why", "what" and "how" and can be a precursor to more detailed research or study. It is generally accepted that case studies are best suited to a "comprehensive, holistic, and in-depth investigation of a complex issue" [26], and as such, this research design was deemed well suited to an examination of CLAN's work to improve health outcomes for children living with CAH in the Asia Pacific region over the last 15 years.

This case study uses the widely accepted Knowledge to Action (KTA) framework [27] developed in 2006 (see Figure 2) to inform and structure analysis. The KTA framework has been acknowledged by the World Health Organisation (WHO) as a useful tool for addressing complex problems in health [28] and facilitates a cohesive summary of the cyclical, PAR nature of CLAN's work over a prolonged period of time. The KTA framework describes a process whereby existing knowledge and insights are augmented by local contextual adaptation, and implementation plans are then informed in a continuous way by existing and emerging insights. In this way, knowledge creation (and ultimately, the products and tools that are developed over time) and knowledge implementation are dynamically inter-linked, both contributing to resolving the "problem" identified as requiring action.

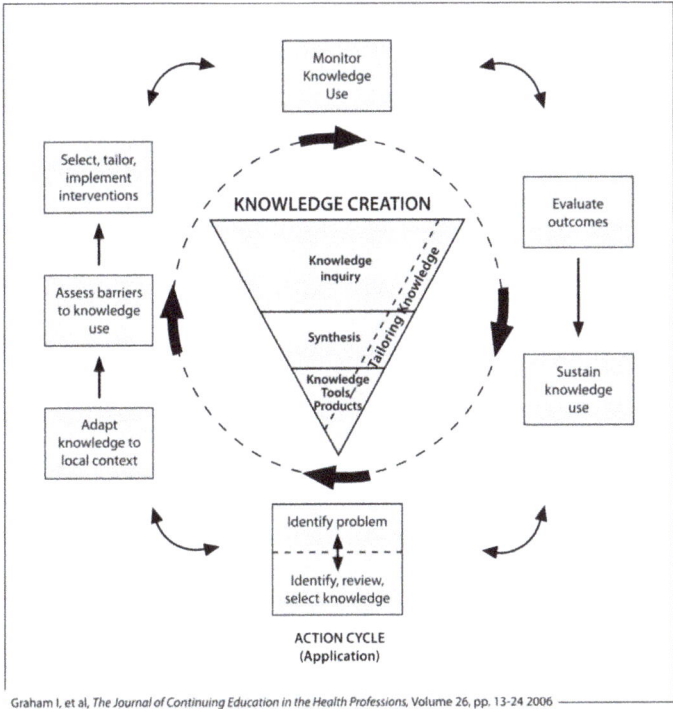

Figure 2. Knowledge to Action (KTA) framework [27] reproduced with permission.

Graham [27] identified seven phases of the action cycle in the KTA framework, and these informed the analysis in this case study by providing an overarching structure to describe how CLAN's model was first developed and then implemented to redress inequities for children living with CAH (and later other chronic health conditions) in the Asia Pacific region between 2004 and 2020.

The seven stages of the KTA framework action cycle are:

1. Identify the problem—identify, review and select knowledge;
2. Adapt knowledge to local context;
3. Assess barriers to knowledge use;
4. Select, tailor and implement interventions;
5. Monitor knowledge use;
6. Evaluate outcomes;
7. Sustain knowledge use.

In line with accepted methods for exploratory case studies [29], the data and evidence informing this paper draw on publicly available material, including: insights from an initial health needs assessment undertaken with the CAH community of Vietnam in 2005 (results published in 2006 [14], with ethics approval having been granted by collaborating institutions in Australia and Vietnam);

published documents (available in peer reviewed and grey literature and referenced accordingly in this article); historical archives (CLAN annual reports, available online [13] and in the National Library of Australia); and conference abstracts.

3. Results

Key activities and historical milestones relating to CLAN's work to support children living with CAH in Vietnam—and, later, in other countries, and with other chronic health conditions—are presented in the context of the seven stages of the KTA framework's action cycle. The subsequent impact of these activities on knowledge creation (notably knowledge inquiry, synthesis and the development of products and tools) is documented also.

3.1. Identify the Problem—Identify, Review and Select Knowledge

Articles and letters in the 2004 CAHSGA (CAH Support Group of Australia) and CARES (CAH Advocacy, Research, Education and Support) Foundation newsletters [30,31] powerfully described some of the inequities experienced by children and families living with CAH in Vietnam.

Michele Konheiser, the Australian mother of a child with CAH travelled to Vietnam with Professor Garry Warne (Paediatric Endocrinologist, Royal Children's Hospital, Melbourne), and wrote:

"I heard stories of parents giving their child one tablet every few days as they couldn't afford daily medication."

"The supply is unreliable. Sometimes they just can't get the medication. The black market can, therefore, charge whatever it likes."

"One lady ... broke down in tears and I found myself in tears as well. She had so much grief inside her."

Prof Warne likewise shared:

"In Vietnam, many parents cannot afford to buy the drugs their children need."

"One bottle of tablets cost the equivalent of 16 bags of rice."

"No 17OHP testing* ... Poor surgical outcomes ... Several deaths annually."

(*Note: a 17OHP blood test measures 17 hydroxyprogesterone and is routinely used in high-income countries for diagnosing and monitoring CAH)

Clearly, the situation described in Vietnam was completely different to that experienced by CAH families in high-income countries at the time—particularly when compared to countries such as Australia, where universal health coverage (UHC—in the form of *Medicare*) [32] ensures essential medicines and quality health care are affordably available to all.

Reflection on the newsletter articles; personal communication with the authors at the time (Michele Konheiser and Garry Warne); personal insight in to the pain of almost losing a child with CAH; and the lived experience of watching a child with CAH who does not receive medicines deteriorate in a relatively short space of time offered (Kate Armstrong) a unique and acute appreciation of the urgent life and death nature of the families' plight.

Access to medicines for all children living with CAH in Vietnam was clearly the most immediate and life-threatening problem. Whilst ever essential medicines (glucocorticoid and mineralocorticoid tablet replacement, and hydrocortisone for injection during acute illness) were neither registered nor affordably available in Vietnam, many children with CAH in Vietnam were at risk of dying from a salt-wasting crisis, and discussions around quality of life became largely irrelevant until this humanitarian crisis could be resolved. Estimates at the time (based on discussions with doctors in Australia and Vietnam) suggested there were approximately 300 children across the whole of Vietnam alive with CAH (hereafter referred to as the *CAH Community of Vietnam*) who would require urgent humanitarian aid until such time as longer-term, sustainable, in-country solutions could be identified.

Direct contact was made (by Kate Armstrong) with two companies in Australia who produced the hydrocortisone tablets (Alphapharm—now Mylan [33]) and fludrocortisone tablets (Bristol-Myers Squibb [34]) used by the CAH Community of Australia. Both companies generously agreed to donate enough hydrocortisone and fludrocotisone tablets for the entire CAH Community of Vietnam for a three-year period, and a commitment was made, through the founding of CLAN, that distribution of these medicines would be securely coordinated over the short-term (three years), whilst longer-term, sustainable solutions were sought in collaboration with local partners [35–37].

3.2. Adapt Knowledge to Local Context

Once access to the essential medicines parents needed to keep their children with CAH alive had been secured, there was a need to consider other priorities and needs of the CAH Community of Vietnam. In this regard, the need for more in depth two-way learning rapidly emerged: CLAN was keen to learn more about the challenges and burdens facing CAH families in Vietnam; and health professionals and families in Vietnam were requesting information and knowledge from Australia that would help children living with CAH in Vietnam achieve the same quality of life and health outcomes people living with CAH in high-income countries of the world were enjoying. There was a need to work together to create and exchange knowledge; as well as share existing (or develop novel) tools and resources that could be used to redress inequities.

With processes for exporting donated drugs to Vietnam established (thanks to generous support from executives of the National Hospital of Pediatrics (NHP) in Hanoi), and mutual agreement reached on the need for strong and transparent systems and partnerships to sustainably facilitate safe delivery of medicines over a three-year period, CLAN received a formal invitation to travel to Vietnam in 2005 to assist with distribution of the medicines, and learn more from local authorities and stakeholders about the best ways to engage moving forward. It was agreed that CLAN would have permission to work in collaboration with health professionals at NHP and Royal Children's Hospital International (RCHI) Melbourne to survey families of children living with CAH and receiving care at NHP (with ethics clearance received from both institutions) so that a shared understanding of the challenges and barriers faced by the CAH Community of Vietnam might inform future collaborative efforts.

There were no existing validated surveys to draw on, so a template was developed de novo by health professionals and families of people living with CAH in Australia and Vietnam. In order to capture a holistic understanding of the challenges families faced, the survey templates included a focus on:

- demographic profiles;
- medication use and purchase;
- routine management of CAH;
- management of adrenal crises;
- health and quality of life;
- specific challenges experienced by girls living with CAH;
- understanding other burdens or questions families might have.

The survey was translated into Vietnamese by a local paediatric endocrinologist, and distributed to families at a CAH Club meeting sponsored by CLAN at NHP on 10 June 2005. The results of this health needs assessment (HNA) were presented back to NHP and the CAH community of Vietnam, as well as published in the Journal of Pediatric Endocrinology and Metabolism in 2006 [14].

Acknowledging locally contextualised insights from the surveys would not be available until after the June 2005 CAH Club meeting, preparation for the Club (patient support group) meeting included efforts to identify and share existing knowledge, tools and resources considered valuable by children and families living with CAH in Australia. A CLAN CAH Club newsletter and PowerPoint presentations were developed and a young person living with CAH in Australia (CH) attended the meeting as part of CLAN's team and co-authored the final paper.

Resources translated into Vietnamese for use by families in advance of the 2005 CAH Club Meeting focused on simple messaging, such as how to optimally use the newly available medicines. There was acknowledgement of the fact hydrocortisone and fludrocortisone tablets had to date been rationed by families, and parents would likely need encouragement to use previously scarce medicines as per the internationally recognized CAH treatment guidelines of the time for routine use (two to three time daily dosing, with triple dosing of hydrocortisone on sick days) [38]. Families were informed of the vital importance of seeking an emergency injection of hydrocortisone from the nearest available health centre to manage adrenal crises if oral hydrocortisone was not sufficient on sick days, and CLAN accepted the advice of local practitioners that it would take time before the Australian practice of ensuring all families had an injection kit at home for use in emergencies could be replicated in Vietnam. Indeed, it took approximately five years before this became common practice, with all families receiving injection kits for the first time at the 2008 CAH Club meetings [39].

As time passed, and the CAH community of Vietnam matured and their knowledge of CAH deepened, more complex educational material was translated into Vietnamese. At the July 2011 CAH Club meeting in Hanoi, the Vietnamese version of C. Y. Hsu and S. A. Rivkees' comprehensive 290-page book *CAH: A Parents' Guide* was launched, and free copies of the book were given to all families attending the Club meetings (260 families attended in Hanoi, and another 100 families attended Club meetings at Children's Hospitals 1 and 2 in Ho Chi Minh City) [40–42]. Free copies of the book were also made available to all hospital executives and health professionals caring for children with CAH, and all other CAH families who were not able to attend the Club meetings for whatever reason.

3.3. Assess Barriers to Knowledge Use

Analysis of responses to the 2005 HNA informed a more detailed understanding of the underlying barriers and challenges experienced by children and families living with CAH in Vietnam at the time.

Families offered insights regarding the impact of:

- Unaffordable and unreliable access to essential medicines—overwhelmingly identified as the most urgent priority.
- Poverty—low incomes (particularly for remote and rural families) were exacerbated by the high cost of medicines and ongoing expenditure and loss of income associated with accessing quality care at tertiary and quaternary centres far from home (few families would trust any health professionals outside of NHP).
- Knowledge and skills gaps—there was an expressed need for education and training on CAH for children, youth, families and health professionals (especially local doctors, who were not considered knowledgeable enough about CAH to manage adrenal crises). Specific queries around genetic counselling and prenatal diagnosis of CAH were also common.
- Language barriers—despite the availability of information on CAH in English, almost all families could only speak Vietnamese, and online translation was not yet readily available.
- Isolation and lack of networks—for both individuals and health professionals.
- Misinformation and myths—were clearly dominant where there was an absence of accurate information.
- Social stigma, beliefs and attitudes—notably cultural considerations, such as fears for children around future marriage and procreation prospects.
- Virilisation—particularly surgical and psycho-social concerns for girls living with CAH when access to medicine had been compromised.
- Health-system challenges for children living with chronic health conditions—such as the complex referral processes, and gaps in existing universal health insurance systems with regards outpatient care for NCDs of childhood.
- Travel and transportation challenges for those living some distance from NHP.

Acknowledging the complexity of the situation, and aligned with a critical realist view of causation [43], a "But why?" root cause analysis (also described as the five whys approach [44]) of these insights was conducted to better understand the *"causes of the causes"* [45] impacting adversely on families of children living with CAH in Vietnam. For instance, medicine was not affordably available.

But why? It was not sold in local pharmacies. But why? It was illegal for pharmacists to sell it. But why? It was not registered in Vietnam. But why? It was not identified as a high priority essential medicine. But why? There were very few children alive with CAH in Vietnam so there was no national focus, and it was not on the WHO Essential Medicines List for children (WHO EMLc) [46] so was not prioritized at an international level. But why? and so on.

This process was continued in some detail, until all of the challenges and barriers had been analysed in depth by CLAN. Emerging from this process was the identification of five key priorities for action (the "five pillars") which have since informed CLAN's model (CLAN's Strategic Framework for Action):

Pillar 1. Access to medicines and equipment—with a focus on solutions that are short-term (e.g., humanitarian aid), medium-term (e.g., registration of drugs nationally) and long-term (inclusion of essential medicines on national insurance lists).

Pillar 2. Access to education, research and advocacy—including translation of educational material; delivery of training; research and advocacy with a view to empowering families, health professionals and the broader community (locally, nationally and internationally).

Pillar 3. Optimisation of medical management—with a holistic, person- and family-centred approach that encompasses primary, secondary and tertiary prevention, and acknowledges the power of multidisciplinary care.

Pillar 4. Encouragement of family support groups—strengthening networks and partnerships to reduce social isolation and empower families, using tertiary and quaternary government/public hospitals as the geographic hub, and families as the visual hub of collaborative action.

Pillar 5. Actions to reduce financial burdens and promote financial independence—encouraging a broad range of initiatives to reduce the financial burden on families and strengthen capacity of future generations to escape poverty (including but not limited to promoting health insurance, attendance at school and vocational training).

Over time, acknowledging the importance of ethical management and processes, CLAN introduced an internal "Pillar 6" that commits the organization to strong governance and accountability mechanisms. To date this has included a commitment to:

- Incorporation as an NGO with the New South Wales (NSW) Department of Fair Trade;
- Fundraising certification with the Office of Liquor and Gaming, NSW;
- Registration with and annual compliance reporting to the Australian Charities and Not-for-Profits Commission (ACNC);
- Signatory to the Code of Conduct and annual Compliance Self Assessment (CSA) audits of the Australian Council For International Development (ACFID) [47];
- Annual reports submitted to the National Library of Australia;
- Tax deductibility status (TDS) and overseas aid gift deductibility status (OAGDS) with the Australian Taxation Office (ATO) and Department of Foreign Affairs and Trade (DFAT);
- Formal association with the United Nations Department of Public Information for NGOs (UNDPI/NGO);
- Special Consultative Status with the UN's Economic and Social Council (ECOSOC); and
- Community of Practice (COP) member status with the World Health Organisation's Non-Communicable Disease Global Coordinating Mechanism (WHO NCD/GCM).

3.4. Select, Tailor and Implement Interventions

In consultation with a range of partners and stakeholders, a collaborative plan for action was developed in light of the 2005 HNA findings. Some of the actions included in this strategic "Plan for CLAN" and actioned over the last 15 years are summarized in Table 1. Not only was this strategic planning document important in terms of promoting transparent communication of priorities and intentions with local authorities, it also facilitated engagement of a broad range of multisectoral stakeholders in collaborative action, enabling a comprehensive, holistic approach to fast tracking change whilst minimising duplication of efforts to redress inequities. Close communication with local health professionals and CAH Club executive members ensured local priorities and real-time feedback informed ongoing activities.

Table 1. Specific examples of tailored, collaborative interventions to support the Congenital Adrenal Hyperplasia (CAH) community in Vietnam.

Priorities	CLAN Activities
Pillar 1. Access to medicines and equipment	*Short-term initiatives* Three year donation of hydrocortisone and fludrocortisone tablets secured; use of hydrocortisone for injection promoted and injection kits shared *Medium term* Hydrocortisone and fludrocortisone tablets registered in Vietnam; rapid assessment protocol completed with the International Insulin Foundation [48] to analyse access to medicines in Vietnam; collaborative application to have hydrocortisone and fludrocortisone tablets included in the World Health Organisation Essential Medicines List for Children (WHO EMLc). *Long term* Essential medicines for CAH included within national insurance scheme
Pillar 2. Education, research and advocacy	*Education* Translation of educational resources into Vietnamese language; educational sessions for health care professionals (HCPs) prior to Club meetings; educational sessions for families/youth at Club meetings (led by local HCPs); training for HCPs both onsite (Australian nurse educator spent 6 months in Vietnam) and in Australia (endocrinologist training in Australia with APPES (the Asia Pacific Pediatric Endocrinology Society)). *Research* Health needs assessment completed and published in journal; RAPIA adapted for CAH and completed in Vietnam [48]; CLAN-APPES Snapshot Survey developed to rapidly identify inequities [15]. *Advocacy* Presentation on CAH activities at APPES Conference; Child-friendly CAH Rights Flyers (raise awareness of the United Nations (UN) Convention on the Rights of the Child using five pillars) [49]; Club newsletters in Vietnamese (include FAQs; latest information on CAH; messages of support from international community) and videos to raise awareness [50]; Club reports (English) shared with all key partners internationally; success stories/videos shared internationally (CLAN website/social media); CLAN panel at 2010 UN Department of Public Information for Non-Government Organisations (UNDPI/NGO) Conference in Melbourne; APPES Declaration 2018 [51].
Pillar 3. Optimisation of medical management	*Primary prevention* Genetic counselling education and training *Secondary prevention* Staff training and education to promote early diagnosis; availability of 17 Hydroxyprogesterone (17OHP) testing for diagnosis and monitoring; newborn screening (NBS) pilot scaled to national program. *Tertiary prevention* Staff and family education and training; educational resources and clinical guidelines available in Vietnamese; affordable access to essential monitoring and equipment (such as 17OHP, renin, genetic testing and injection kits); support for gynaecology and surgical teams to exchange internationally [52]; and promotion of growth charts for routine monitoring. *Holistic care* Strengthened focus on patient and family centred care; training in psychological support; information about pregnancy for people living with CAH.
Pillar 4. Encourage Support Groups	Support of annual Club meetings; CAH Club executive nominated; communication networks established (Facebook, Whats App, Twitter, Instagram); connections with international CAH support networks facilitated; training sessions facilitated for families and health professionals; success stories from international CAH Communities shared to inspire.
Pillar 5. Reduce financial burdens	Children encouraged to attend school; awards for school performance; education on emergency management/injection kits reduce need to travel; medicine affordably available (on national insurance scheme) and facilitation of international supply chains to optimise pricing; systematic outpatient care (reduce travel and unapproved expenses).
Pillar 6. Ethical & transparent management	CLAN incorporated as non-governmental organisation in Australia [13]; fundraising certification; ethical governance and accountability processes; multilateral engagement, reporting and accountability.

Maintaining the national "community of children living with CAH in Vietnam" as a visual hub was key to promoting a shared, person-centred mission amongst all stakeholders. With children and families central to all discussions, a sustained focus on shared goals (redressing inequities and improving health outcomes) was achieved. With access to essential medicines secured early (Pillar 1), it was possible to focus limited resources and collective action on other pillars. Translation of educational resources and development of specific tools and resources, such as informational videos in Vietnamese and a Club newsletter (Pillar 2); facilitation of professional development opportunities for staff (Pillar 3); and fundraising to support Club meetings (Pillars 4 and 6) were able to occur in parallel. All such actions ultimately helped reduce financial burdens on families (Pillar 5), until such time as real change was achieved through the profound commitments by the Vietnamese government to implement nation-wide policy changes (such as the inclusion of both hydrocortisone and fludrocortisone on the national essential medicines and insurance list; and implementation of NBS for CAH) which have ultimately had the most profoundly transformational impact on the lives of the CAH Community.

3.5. Monitor Knowledge Use

In accordance with CLAN's internal "sixth pillar", timely monitoring, evaluation and reporting have been central to efforts to drive change for children living with CAH in Vietnam and beyond.

Reflecting CLAN's commitment to continuous quality improvement (CQI), indicators used to monitor and evaluate the use of knowledge at the individual, health professional and systems levels are numerous (see Table A1) and include measures of:

1. Conceptual knowledge use—this includes changes in levels of knowledge, understanding or attitudes. Examples of indicators used to monitor knowledge use included: the CAH PepTalk Tool [53], developed to evaluate parental knowledge of CAH and its management; numbers of families and health professionals attending Club meetings and training sessions (reflected degree of engagement); nature of questions posed by families at Club meetings (a useful barometer of the general understanding of the community and tool for identifying widely held myths and misunderstandings); engagement of external partners and stakeholders; and requests to CLAN to scale CAH activities to other hospitals (in Vietnam and beyond) and health conditions.
2. Instrumental knowledge use—monitors changes in behavior or practice (and most importantly, changes that translate into improved health outcomes). Examples of indicators used included: availability and registration of drugs (reflecting the broader health system); use of injection kits on sick days at home by families; patient registers tracking incidence, prevalence, mortality and loss to follow-up; use of growth charts (introduced for routine use in outpatient clinics); availability and quality of educational resources in local language for families and health professionals; availability and analysis of 17OHP and renin testing; use of genetic analysis; and establishment of NBS for CAH.
3. Strategic knowledge use—is the manipulation of knowledge to attain specific power or profit goals (sometimes referred to as "research as ammunition"). Examples of indicators included: publication of results and presentations at international conferences; collaborative engagement in civil society networks; engagement with multilaterals and member state governments; participation of media at Club meetings; requests received to translate CLAN's model to other conditions and countries; and the number and types of communities established internationally.

In 2015 CLAN collaborated with members of the Asia Pacific Pediatric Endocrinology Society (APPES) [54] to undertake the APPES-CLAN Equity (ACE) "Snapshot Survey", which provided a rapid landscape analysis of the situation for children living with CAH and three other key endocrine conditions (type 1 diabetes, OI and congenital hypothyroidism (CH)) across the Asia Pacific region with regards to many of the indicators listed above. This consultation process helped to rapidly identify vulnerable communities of children and activities that could be realistically and affordably implemented to improve quality of life for those most at risk, and informed the 2016 Tokyo Declaration (formally approved by APPES Council, November 2016), which acknowledges the inequities facing children living with paediatric endocrine conditions in the Asia Pacific region, and endorses a collective commitment to advocacy, action and sustainable change [51,55].

CLAN's annual reports (from 2005 to the present) routinely shared key success stories according to the five pillars and planned action model, and ensured all stakeholders were appropriately acknowledged and updated not only on their own important contributions, but how these were further complemented by the generosity and expertise of others. In this way, awareness of the contributions and achievements of other stakeholders served to encourage not only CAH Communities, but also allowed all stakeholders to share an understanding of their own particular contributions to a movement that was achieving sustainable, long-term change for children living in vulnerable circumstances.

3.6. Evaluate Outcomes—Impact of Using the Knowledge

CLAN is committed to ongoing monitoring and evaluation, as well as reporting back to key stakeholders in a timely manner. In summarising the impact of collaborative efforts to optimize quality of life for children living with CAH in Vietnam and the Asia Pacific region using CLAN's model, the RE-AIM Framework [56] provides a useful structure, and considers: Reach; Efficacy; Adoption; Implementation and Maintenance.

The *Reach* of CLAN's model has been substantial. In Vietnam, CLAN was proud to support CAH Club meetings at the four major children's hospitals in Vietnam over a 10-year period. Engagement of families at these Club meetings grew annually, and within several years quality educational resources (booklets on CAH in Vietnamese) had effectively been shared with almost 100% of children diagnosed with CAH in the country thanks to the strong partnerships established in Hanoi, Ho Chi Minh City and Hue. Essential diagnostic tests were made affordably available in the tertiary hospitals (such as 17OHP and renin testing), and growth charts introduced for routine use in monitoring. Rapid increases in prevalence after 2005 led to the expansion of a pilot NBS trial in 2006, which has since been expanded across Vietnam. Translation of CLAN's model to type 1 diabetes (2007) and osteogenesis imperfecta (2011) helped raise the profile of paediatric endocrinology as a medical specialty in Vietnam, and the Vietnamese Pediatric Endocrinology Society was established shortly afterwards. Members of the Vietnamese Pediatric Endocrinology Society now actively engage and lead in regional and international professional meetings, and publish on CAH and diabetes in peer review journals [53,57–61].

Beyond Vietnam, CLAN received a series of requests for collaboration from paediatric endocrinologists for CAH communities in the Philippines (2005), Indonesia (2006) and Pakistan (2007), whereupon the same model of community development was replicated in each country, with local adaptations as appropriate. Access to medicines was a universal challenge for each country initially, and the collaborative efforts to apply for hydrocortisone and fludrocortisone tablets to be included in the WHO EMLc in 2008 was an important step in driving change internationally. All four countries have since seen improvements in access to essential medicines for their CAH communities to varying degrees. For some countries local production and availability of low cost medicines has been achieved (such as hydrocortisone tablets in Indonesia and Pakistan), whilst in others (such as Vietnam), national registration and importation from affordable, quality suppliers have been the preferred solution.

The *Efficacy* of collaborative efforts to date is perhaps best reflected in the achievements seen at local levels of and for CAH communities in the different countries CLAN has worked.

3.6.1. Vietnam

The prevalence of CAH has increased nationally, with an estimated increase from 150 children at NHP in Hanoi in 2004 to 1235 cases (325 with genotyping completed) in 2018 [62], representing a 723% increase over 14 years. Vietnam's national NBS program now includes CAH (together with congenital hypothyroidism, glucose-6-phosphate dehydrogenase deficiency, galactosemia, phenylketonuria and other inborn errors of metabolism) and has determined the incidence of CAH in Vietnam at 1:9008 live births [63]. Successful implementation of NBS for CAH will continue to strengthen CAH gender equity in Vietnam thanks to early diagnosis and increased survival of males with salt wasting CAH. Molecular diagnosis assists with genetic counselling, and is strengthening diagnostic capacity [64]. A recent publication from Vietnam on genetic analysis of 212 people living with CAH reported six novel variants [62].

Quality of life for the CAH Community in Vietnam is a research priority. Within a few years of the 2005 HNA and sustained actions around the five pillars of CLAN, there were anecdotal reports from local health professionals indicating fewer children were presenting in adrenal crisis; likewise, families shared stories at Club meetings of their experiences using hydrocortisone injections at home on sick days to save their children's lives. Reductions in mortality had an impact on the age profile of the CAH Community: in 2006 only 7% of all children attending NHP for management of CAH were over the age of 13 years [65], but in 2020 detailed follow up on health outcomes for the community are well underway. Formal analysis of quality of life (using the Health-related Quality of Life in Children PedsQL™ 4.0 measurement model [66]) has been completed with 137 children, and a review of clinical health outcomes on a cohort of 81 children at NHP over the age of 10 years includes measures of growth, body mass index, insulin levels, HOMA-IR (homeostatic model assessment of insulin resistance) and metabolic syndrome criteria [63].

A key concern of parents and young people living with CAH shared during CAH Club meetings over the years related to cultural considerations, and in particular, community fears regarding the impact of CAH on potential marriage and child-bearing prospects for young girls later in life. In 2012, CLAN shared a video in Vietnamese language with messaging from an Australian woman living with CAH who had gone on to have children of her own, and this was very well received by the community [67]. In 2020 there are 10 women with CAH treated from childhood at NHP who have now married and had babies of their own [63].

3.6.2. The Philippines

Whilst newborn screening for CAH had been available nationally since 1996, when CLAN was first approached by paediatric endocrinologists from Manila in 2005, neither hydrocortisone nor fludrocortisone tablets were registered or affordably available in country. Short-term humanitarian donations were required for the estimated cohort of 80 children living with CAH in the Philippines at the time (118 children had been diagnosed by NBS as at January 2008) [68], until sustainable local registration and distribution systems were secured.

CLAN attended the inaugural CAH support group meeting for the CAH Community of the Philippines (CAHSAPI) at the Philippines General Hospital's (PGH) Pediatric Department on 11 December 2005, and was proud to support an initial three year donation of hydrocortisone tablets (again, with generous support from Mylan). This humanitarian aid occurred in parallel to a range of community development initiatives, including the translation of educational resources in to Tagalog and annual face-to-face CAHSAPI meetings. CAHSAPI members continue to actively engage with one another on Facebook (established in December 2010 by Mr Alain Yap, the founding president of CAHSAPI), with strong support from paediatric endocrinology staff at PGH, and currently has approximately 280 members [69]—many of them now teenagers. As at December 2017 the number of children diagnosed with CAH through NBS in the Philippines was 576 (1:18,083 of the 10,415,695 infants screened) [70].

3.6.3. Indonesia

Since CLAN first sent emergency humanitarian supplies of hydrocortisone and fludrocortisone tablets to colleagues in Surabaya (and shortly afterwards, all children living with CAH in the country for a three year period in total) following a request for support in 2006, much has changed for children living with CAH in Indonesia.

In 2007, the inaugural Indonesian CAH support group (IKAHAK) started in Surabaya and in 2008 IKAHAK helped to establish a national CAH community called KAHAKI. Collaborative efforts by CLAN, Indonesian paediatric endocrinologists, IKAHAK and KAHAKI focused on securing longer-term, affordable access to essential medications for the CAH community members. Following the inclusion of hydrocortisone and fludrocortisone tablets in the WHO's EMLc in 2008 [68], members of the pediatric endocrinology working group of the Indonesian Pediatric Society began working closely with Indofarma, an Indonesian government-owned pharmaceutical company, regarding the possibility of local hydrocortisone production. Indofarma committed to produce hydrocortisone, however significant time was needed to navigate complex internal factors at Indofarma and other bureaucratic issues. In the interim, medication continued to be sourced in various ways, including from other countries such as the Netherlands, Singapore and Australia to fulfil the ongoing needs of children with CAH. Finally, in 2018, hydrocortisone (Genison) was made available in the market. Hydrocortisone by injection (Fartison) was also produced by a local company in the same year, although fludrocortisone tablets are still not manufactured nationally. One of the drug companies is willing to build a factory to produce fludrocortisone in Indonesia, but efforts have been so far hindered by the COVID-19 pandemic.

In the first year (2009) of the official CAH Registry of the Indonesian Pediatric Society, 69 children were registered (56 females (81%) and 13 males (19%)). This number expanded rapidly, with 439 patients (303 females (69%) and 136 males (31%)) registered in 2020, representing a 536% increase over 11 years. The increase in male patients over this period (from 13 in 2009 to 136 in 2020) represents a 946% increase, which was more than double the rate of change for females (there was a 441% increase in females registered; from 56 in 2009, to 303 in 2020) and may reflect increasing awareness amongst physicians in Indonesia of CAH beyond recognition of ambiguous genitalia in females.

Mortality associated with CAH in Indonesia has reduced over the years, but still represents a significant and preventable inequity. Data reported in Central Java, Indonesia in 2016 indicated ten (13%) of the 78 patients registered with CAH in Central Java since 2009 had died due to adrenal crises. Also of concern, only four (5%) of the 78 patients were male, which may indicate adrenal crises were still going undiagnosed and unidentified in this region at that time [71].

Translation of educational resources on CAH into Bahasa Indonesian has been a collective endeavour, and a locally developed video [72] and booklet specifically addressing the challenges facing teenage girls living with CAH in Indonesia [73] have been very powerful. Emergency cards for families to carry, with instructions written in Bahasa Indonesian have also been available to families since 2019. KAHAKI members use WhatsApp as a tool to communicate with each other, and families use this forum to share their experiences living with CAH, as well as practical tips—such as how to access fludrocortisone tablets.

3.6.4. Pakistan

Communication between CLAN and health professionals at the National Institute of Child Health (NICH) in Pakistan commenced in 2007. Urgent humanitarian donations of hydrocortisone and fludrocortisone tablets were arranged for the estimated 80 children living with CAH in Pakistan at the time, with annual CAH Club meetings culminating in the establishment of CLIP (CAH Living In Pakistan). Key achievements with and for CLIP have included: reduced mortality and loss to follow-up (there are currently 334 receiving care for CAH at NICH alone); collaboration on the WHO EMLc application for inclusion of hydrocortisone and fludrocortisone tablets [74,75]; translation of educational resources on CAH into Urdu; paediatric endocrinology training for local health professionals; support for establishment of SPED (the Society of Pediatric Endocrinology and Diabetes in Pakistan) [76]; development of the SPED app for health professionals (currently has 107 registered health professionals, and provides access to a range of materials to assist with optimization of medical management); and establishment of child psychiatry services. A short-term grant from Pfizer Australia [77] in 2016 enabled CLAN to initiate the employment of a community development officer (CDO) at NICH, which continues to this day and has proven an effective model for facilitating activities around the five pillars [78].

In 2020 two particularly encouraging developments have been achieved. Firstly, local production of hydrocortisone tablets (CortiCort 10mg produced by Tabros Pharma) in Pakistan at affordable prices has commenced (Rs: 2.2/tablet; AUD: 0.018/tablet). Secondly, a pilot project funded by CLAN and APPES has trialed the delivery of essential medicines to the homes of 50 CAH community members identified as living in the most vulnerable circumstances (those families living in poverty and/or remote/rural were eligible). This practical step towards improving access to essential medicines for children living in the most disadvantaged circumstances has already proven very effective, with near universal compliance and follow-up achieved with all fifty children throughout the COVID-19 pandemic a remarkable outcome.

Since 2004 *Adoption* of CLAN's model has occurred in more than 10 countries and has been used to address over 10 different NCDs of childhood, thereby demonstrating its adaptability across a wide variety of conditions, cultures, languages, healthcare and political systems.

CLAN does not actively seek new partners to adopt its model. In the early years, positive messaging around CLAN's work initially spread by word of mouth, with paediatric endocrinologists in the Asia Pacific region communicating directly with one another through their professional networks (notably APPES) on the changes they were seeing for the children and families they cared for. Individual health professionals would approach CLAN privately asking if the model could be replicated in their own setting.

As awareness of CLAN's achievements grew (through sharing of success stories, tools and resources on CLAN's website, publications and conference presentations globally) direct requests for assistance would also come from families of children living with CAH and other chronic health conditions in resource-poor settings. In these instances, CLAN would encourage families and health professionals to connect locally and nationally to collaborate jointly with CLAN and other stakeholders to scale change in systematic and sustainable ways. CLAN always made it clear that our focus was on community development: CLAN does not export medicines to families or health professionals where individual patients are the sole recipients (the only exception to this being situations where only one or two children with a particular condition are known to be alive in a country, as was the case in Fiji for Osteogenesis Imperfecta in 2016).

In this regard, a vitally important step in commencing work with new partners in any country, or for any chronic condition of childhood, is to communicate clearly the foundational principles that inform every aspect of CLAN's work. The principles inform CLAN's approach to implementing our strategic framework for action and the five pillars, and include:

1. A holistic view of health—CLAN acknowledges the WHO definition of health [79], with a focus on body, mind and spirit, and an appreciation of the impact the socio-cultural determinants of health (SCDOH) [45] have on health outcomes.
2. Human rights-based approach—acknowledging rights and responsibilities as outlined in the United Nations' Convention on the Rights of the Child [80].
3. Equity—a commitment to strive for excellence for all, and ensuring the rights of children in high- and low-income countries to the highest quality of life possible are respected, promoted and protected.
4. Community development—all children living with the same chronic health condition in a country are members of a community; these NCD Communities are considered as interconnected and united at the local, regional, national and international level.
5. Community control—people living with chronic conditions are experts and must be consulted at all stages when decisions are made around appropriate approaches and actions to drive change.
6. Person- and family-centred care—acknowledges the pivotal role children, young people and families play in all activities. Indeed, a number of parents of children with chronic health

conditions have stayed engaged with CLAN over a decade, and have been champions in their country for change.
7. Sustainable, ethical and transparent approaches to project management—CLAN is committed to the highest standards of accountability and reporting required of NGOs (by ACFID) in Australia and to the United Nations (through UNDPI/NGO and ECOSOC); as a not-for-profit CLAN is committed to sustainable approaches and responsible action in the face of climate change.
8. Multisectoral collaboration and partnerships—are key to sustainability and success.
9. Above all do no harm—is an overarching guiding principle and informs all actions.

To date, key learnings from work with CAH Communities in the Asia Pacific (and later Nigeria in 2012) have since been transferred to support children living with:

- Type 1 diabetes—Vietnam (2007), Pakistan (2007) and Indonesia (2020);
- Osteogenesis imperfecta (OI)—Vietnam (2011), Indonesia (2013), Pakistan (2014) and Fiji (2016);
- Duchenne muscular dystrophy (DMD)—Vietnam (2012);
- Nephrotic syndrome (NS)—Vietnam (2010);
- Rheumatic heart disease (RHD)—Kenya (2013);
- Nodding syndrome and epilepsy—Uganda (2017);
- Thalassaemia—India (2020);
- Asthma, cancer, autism and cerebral palsy (amongst others)—collaborative advocacy efforts in multiple countries.

CLAN's model has been validated across conditions, countries, cultures and communities, achieving comparable outcomes and positive impacts in a diverse range of settings. Co-design and local adaptation have always been a feature of *Implementation* of the model, and integral to the successful outcomes and impact seen. CAH communities in different countries had different starting points, so individual national strategic plans had to be developed each time.

One clear indicator of local ownership is often the names chosen by the communities CLAN has worked with across the Asia Pacific region. For instance, CAH Communities we partner with include: CAHSAPI in the Philippines (the name includes a play on the Tagalog word "kasapi" meaning "being a member or part of"); IKAHAK and KAHAKI (a play on words and sounds using "KAH" for CAH in Bahasa Indonesian); and CLIP in Pakistan (an acronym for *CAH Living in Pakistan*). CLAN's commitment to community development is strengthened by our sixth pillar's guidance around ethical and transparent management, and our long-term compliance to the rigorous self-assessment and reporting requirements of full signatories to ACFID's code of conduct reflects this. Whilst the cost benefits of CLAN's model have not been formally evaluated by health economists, the engagement and uptake of the model (usually for more than one condition in each country) suggests local authorities see value in any implementation costs.

Sustainability is a foundational principle for CLAN's model, and the need for *Maintenance* of efforts over the longer-term is acknowledged as fundamental to success. That said, whilst some of CLAN's original stakeholders and partners are no longer actively engaged, this is not necessarily always a negative outcome. For instance, humanitarian donations of hydrocortisone and fludrocortisone are no longer urgently needed in most of the countries CLAN has worked in due to successful efforts by governments, local health professionals and community members to secure longer term, sustainable localized solutions. By contrast, long-term engagement of other stakeholders over the years speaks to the success of CLAN's model, and particularly in the case of relationships with the CAH Club executive and leaders, indicates the importance of engaging parents and young people living with CAH and other NCDs, given the chronic, life-long nature of most NCDs.

Social media and technology (notably Facebook, WhatsApp, SMS messaging and websites) have proven a cost-effective vehicle for maintaining connections and raising awareness, and are certainly pivotal to maintaining networks amongst young people and families living with CAH in resource-poor communities of the Asia Pacific region. Introductions between CAH Club Members in Vietnam and other international CAH support group networks (notably, Australia, New Zealand, UK, USA, Philippines, Indonesia and Pakistan) strengthen a sense of international belonging and community, as well as opportunities for sharing updates, information and support. International awareness days (such as Wishbone Day [81] for the OI Community on 6 May each year) have proven powerful platforms for community development activities.

3.7. Sustain Knowledge Use

In additional to local action, CLAN has always committed to ensuring community priorities and voices inform international advocacy and efforts to raise awareness of the challenges facing children and young people who are living not just with CAH, but rather NCDs more generally. To this end, CLAN was proud to serve as the inaugural Secretariat of NCD Child [82], with a view to promoting the voices of children and adolescents within the international NCD discourse. Early achievements of the NCD Child movement included acknowledgement of children, young people and a life course approach to NCDs within the 2011 UN High Level Meeting Declaration on NCDs [83]; and acknowledgement at the 2013 World Health Assembly that *"(c)hildren can die from treatable non-communicable diseases, such as rheumatic heart disease, type 1 diabetes, asthma, and leukaemia, if health promotion, disease prevention, and comprehensive care are not provided"* (page 8, para 2 [84]). These seemingly simple statements were the first time chronic conditions of childhood had been acknowledged by member states and the WHO in the context of the global NCD discourse, and now offer a powerful platform for future advocacy and negotiation by NCD community members, health professionals and health system officials.

CLAN has continued to engage as a participant in the WHO's Global Coordinating Mechanism (GCM) on NCDs since transitioning from the Secretariat role of NCD Child in 2014, and more recently has proudly taken on the role of inaugural Secretariat for IndigenousNCDs [85], a movement committed to privileging First Nations voices on the issue of NCDs. CLAN's rights-based, community development approach seeks to strengthen the capacity of First Nations peoples to advocate for action that addresses the especial inequitable burdens experienced by their children, young people and other community members living with chronic health conditions, too often in resource poor settings.

A consideration of cost is relevant here, and it is important to note CLAN is a not a large NGO, and in fact when assessed according to ACFID criteria ranks amongst the smallest NGOs in Australia. Relying on volunteers and modest donations and grants, CLAN's commitment to cost-effective sustainable solutions comes as much from necessity as it does from choice. More than ever, high-impact, low-cost initiatives such as publications, social media and website use, networking and collaboration with like-minded organisations will be key to success and sustainability. Whilst annual support group meetings provide the perfect vehicle for early support and longer term engagement, as access to medicine is secured locally, online platforms are established and locally developed tools, products and resources are utilised, the subsequent baseline knowledge, expertise and connectedness of the CAH community and their local health professionals strengthens, thereby reducing reliance on international partners for support.

4. Discussion

4.1. Limitations and Challenges

It is important to acknowledge there are limitations to the extent to which persons directly involved in or collaborating with the work of CLAN can objectively evaluate the benefits and merit of activities, much less their outcome and impact. Analysis of CLAN's model using the KTA framework was an attempt to bring some objectivity to the process of describing the work of CLAN and how we have worked with others to overcome the many challenges and burdens facing children living with CAH and other NCDs in resource-poor settings. The authors note more research in this field is urgently needed. Cohort studies and randomized controlled trials with chronic conditions of childhood such as

CAH are extremely limited and rarely population based, therefore the data in this report are based on the KTA framework and CLAN's model rather than more rigorous study designs. Future research could include comparative studies in countries using CLAN's framework versus those who are not.

Financing for NCDs globally is a major challenge, and there is increasing recognition of the inequitable burden carried by the poorest peoples living in the poorest countries with NCDs such as CAH [86]. To complicate this further, it is not just the poor who are impoverished by NCDs. CLAN's experience has been that even relatively wealthy families of children living in countries where quality care is not affordably available risk bankruptcy over time, gradually selling all their assets and ultimately joining the ranks of the "poorest billion" as a result of catastrophic health spends in (too often futile) attempts to save their loved one. With this in mind, it is not surprising that chronic underfunding and limited human and material resources are ubiquitous and sustained challenges facing CLAN and other partners working in this space. Encouragingly, experiences over the last 15 years in multiple countries demonstrate innovative approaches which place NCD communities as the central focus of collaborative action have the potential to scale change at national levels for entire populations of children living with chronic conditions in resource poor settings. Investing in communities brings sustainability, and communities themselves are ideally placed to advise on the best ways to strengthen health systems from the grassroots through to the quaternary levels.

Sadly, despite the best efforts, the reality is some lives cannot be saved. In low- and high-resource settings alike, it is imperative humane processes are in place to support families experiencing the trauma of losing their child in the end stages of a chronic health condition (for example cancer or chronic kidney disease). In such circumstances, clear information, supportive health professionals and quality palliative care are needed to reduce the suffering of children and their families alike, and protect parents from their well-intentioned allocation of limited remaining time and funds to chasing elusive cures and expensive therapies that have no evidence base.

4.2. Recommendations

Key recommendations emerging from this case study that are offered to others keen to redress inequities for childhood NCD communities would include:

4.3. Affordable Access to Essential Medicines and Equipment Is Pillar 1 for a Reason

Over many years CLAN's experience has been that humanitarian donations of essential medicines to keep children alive must be the first priority. Much like Maslow's hierarchy of needs [87], affordable access to essential medicines is the foundation on which all future achievements can be built. Whilst it usually takes at least three years of humanitarian donations to keep children alive until local solutions are established, once medicines are affordably available long-term, families are able to focus on thriving, not just surviving.

With local production of affordable, quality hydrocortisone and fludrocortisone now underway in the Asia Pacific region, and both medicines on the WHO EMLc since 2008, there is no justification for any country of the world to deny children living with CAH their basic human rights to life and health. It must be noted here that this is equally the case for insulin, which, some 100 years after its discovery is still unavailable because it is unaffordable to virtually all children and young people living with Type 1 diabetes in low-, middle- and sometimes even high-income countries, such that WHO is now implementing innovative action to increase access globally [88].

4.4. Share the Wheel—Don't Reinvent It

Many health professionals have reached out to CLAN over the years to ask "how does it work" and "can you help?". Whilst CLAN's strategic framework for action speaks clearly to the "who" (NCD community, multisectoral stakeholders) and the "what" (the five pillars) of CLAN's work, the three dimensional model that emerged from this case study (Figure 3—representing the interplay between CLAN's Strategic Framework for Action and the KTA framework) will hopefully prove a more useful tool for communicating the "how" (local adaptation, tailored interventions, participatory action research approaches, sharing of products and tools etc.) of CLAN's model to others in future so that efforts can be taken to scale.

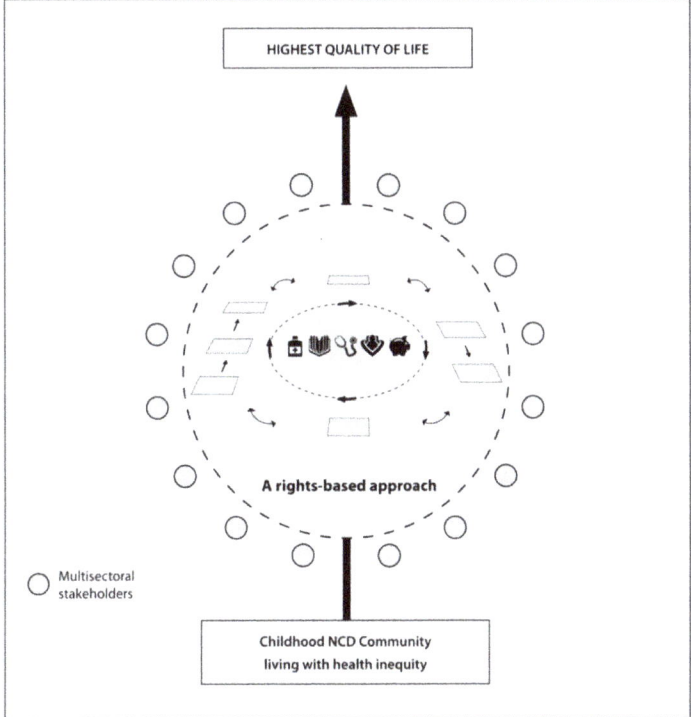

Figure 3. Interplay between CLAN's Strategic Framework for Action and the KTA framework.

CLAN is committed to freely sharing all products, tools and success stories with others so that achievements can be replicated without the need for CLAN to be directly involved. All products and tools referred to in this document (see Table A2 for more details) are available to share, and CLAN acknowledges the many other NGOs working globally to support children living with NCDs and other chronic health conditions. It has been CLAN's experience through the work of NCD Child and IndigenousNCDs that there is almost universal willingness of NGOs in this space to generously share with others so that children everywhere might benefit.

4.5. Community Is Core to Sustainability

On reflection, it is a remarkable achievement for a small NGO to still be operating internationally more than 15 years after the first flash of inspiration. Although a true appreciation of the inherent risks of CLAN's model was not immediately apparent when CLAN was founded, it certainly became clear over time that the very nature of CLAN's vision and mission potentially exposed the organization to inherent risk: a rights-based focus on children living with chronic health conditions in resource-poor settings commits CLAN to working with communities who are amongst the most poor, most inequitably burdened, least powerful and least privileged people in the world.

Ironically however, the reverse outcome has been observed. The inherent strengths, commitment, dedication and resilience of these same communities—those labelled *"poorest of the poor"*—has ultimately underpinned CLAN's greatest successes over time. Of all the stakeholders CLAN has worked with, it is not infrequently the parents of children living with CAH (and later, once conditions improve in a country, young people themselves living with the chronic health condition [65]) with whom we engage most deeply and for the longest periods of time—most usually in their roles as support group executives. For parents of children (and young people themselves) living with the chronic health condition in question, there is a very strong motivation to engage, learn and do what they can to achieve optimal quality of life. There is no question that parents of children living with chronic health conditions in low- and high-income settings alike are almost universally driven by their profound love for their children and sheer determination to do all they can to help their children survive and thrive. The only difference for families in low and high-income settings is the resources and power they have available to them to drive change.

For this reason, when families in resource-poor settings find themselves supported by caring health professionals and other committed partners and stakeholders to redress inequities, they demonstrate time and again a near limitless capacity to contribute to collaborative efforts in very meaningful and deeply committed ways. It is not unusual for CLAN to have worked with some of the same families for over a decade, and this longevity fundamentally impacts on the sustainability of CLAN's model. In this regard, the importance of maintaining communities of children as the visual hub of multisectoral action cannot be over-emphasised.

On that note, NBS programmes may offer a timely opportunity to systematically integrate and promote CLAN's community development approach. The diagnosis of a serious, lifelong condition in a newborn baby is almost invariably a traumatic experience for parents, and particularly in resource-poor settings, systematic and early introductions of these families to the relevant NCD Community networks, tools and resources needed to address the five pillars would impact positively on health outcomes and quality of life for individual children. Moreover, a shared commitment internationally to community networks, growth and well-being within the context of national NBS programmes could be a powerful step towards achieving sustained, collaborative action to address inequities for many childhood NCD communities of the world.

4.6. Knowledge Is Power

Whilst knowledge creation, and the development of products and tools are important, the real key to redressing inequities is knowledge exchange. We must tailor knowledge to action and action to knowledge, tools and products if we are to strengthen community health literacy. There is already ample evidence available from a variety of settings (high- and low-income alike) regarding the best ways to optimize quality of life for children living with chronic health conditions such as CAH; the real challenge is to translate and localize this knowledge to action in resource-poor settings so that no child is left behind.

Where language is a barrier to accessing knowledge from other community settings, specific efforts must be made to translate material into locally and culturally appropriate resources [89]. Families and health professionals alike require detailed, "deep" knowledge to effectively manage complex chronic health conditions, so although simple, easy to read resources are satisfactory in the short term, over the longer term more comprehensive educational resources for families and health professionals alike should be a major priority. Raising awareness amongst communities of their children's basic human rights to health and life [80]—and the responsibilities others in society have to protect and promote same—is a core component of CLAN's work, and our child-friendly rights flyers (available in a range of languages) have been designed to assist with this [49].

4.7. Two-Way Learning Strengthens Us All

For those with the capacity for and interest in action, the rationale for involvement need not be simply altruistic. For stakeholders in low-income countries, the cost-benefit of investing in the lives of children and young people who are living with, and at risk of NCDs, can be enormous. Childhood offers a "golden window" of opportunity in the developmental trajectory of future generations, and simple innovations can pay great dividends. For families and health professionals in high-income countries, there is much to learn from our counterparts in resource poor settings and the potential for, and benefits of, two-way learning must not be understated. For instance, Vietnam is now leading the way in genetic analysis for CAH, and has much to offer children, families and health professionals living in Australia and other high-income countries with their expertise in this field. Colleagues in Pakistan are leading the way in the development of mobile phone applications that can provide critical clinical information to health care professionals and service large numbers of families at low cost; and Pakistani pharmaceutical companies are now producing affordable, quality essential medicines for CAH. The Philippines has world class expertise in NBS that many others can learn from, and Indonesia's innovative educational resources fill informational gaps [90]. A strengths-based approach to collaborative partnerships and two-way learning pays huge dividends for all.

4.8. Prioritise Children and Families Experiencing the Greatest Inequities

Knowing where to focus energies to redress inequities can be a challenge. Whilst CLAN has to date responded to requests for assistance where communities and health professionals self-identify urgent concerns, a more systematic approach to identifying those childhood NCD communities most in need of action should be a global priority. Current United Nations Sustainable Development Goals [91] have a limited focus on preventable morbidity and mortality relating to NCDs in children and young people, and this represents a major opportunity for future knowledge creation and action. Investment in taking the APPES-CLAN Equity (ACE) Snapshot Survey to scale may enable rapid identification of communities most in need of urgent action.

4.9. Embrace Imperfection amongst Complexity

Whilst the action needed to redress inequities associated with childhood NCDs and other chronic health conditions is not necessarily expensive, it does take time and commitment from a broad range of stakeholders. Holistic, comprehensive approaches are essential. There is never a single easy quick fix, but this should neither paralyse nor prevent us from making a start—a critical realist perspective encourages us that even an imperfect start is better than nothing.

On that note—a bit like *do-re-mi* in the Sound of Music [92]—the five pillars of CLAN provide a very good place to start. Whilst a locally adapted approach is the gold standard, CLAN's experiences over multiple conditions, countries and cultures have proved to us again and again that stakeholders can be confident action plans developed around the five pillars will set them on the right path until such time as a deeper understanding of local context is achieved. As the song concludes *"Once you know the notes to sing, you can sing most anything"*, so it is with the five pillars of CLAN when tackling complex chronic health conditions of childhood.

That said, realistic expectations are of course essential. CLAN's model speaks to continuous, long-term approaches. Change will not happen overnight. At least, not until it does.

By way of example, COVID-19—the disease caused by the severe acute respiratory syndrome coronavirus 2 (SARS-CoV-2)—brings new challenges, particularly as the virus presents the greatest risk to people with existing health conditions [93], such that special efforts must be made to ensure the rights of children and young people living with NCDs in both high- and low-income settings are protected and promoted throughout this pandemic. Fragile essential medicine supply chains, over-burdened health systems and financial devastation of families in resource poor settings present real and especial risk to the families CLAN has worked with over many years. Ongoing commitment to equity and health for all will be essential if hard-earned gains are to be maintained. The World Bank estimates COVID-19 will push between 71 and 100 million people into extreme poverty [94] and initiatives ensuring future vaccines go to those who need it, not just to those who can afford it [95], are especially relevant in the case of children living with chronic health conditions in resource-poor settings. Whilst unexpected challenges can be incorporated within the cyclical approach of the KTA and CLAN frameworks, sustained and proactive steps are required by a range of stakeholders to redress inequities. It is essential to maintain flexibility at all times, such that activities and project plans can be rapidly tailored and adapted in real time to adapt to novel circumstances. The scale of some challenges can seem over-whelming at times, but when we work together, and seek collectively to prioritise those living in the most vulnerable circumstances, it is possible to make a difference.

5. Conclusions

This exploratory case study of CLAN's model using the KTA Framework to inform analysis provides practical insights into the real-life actions that can be taken to tackle a complex health problem such as CAH in resource-poor settings, and positively impact on the lives of entire communities of children and families. Until such time as quality health care and affordable access to medicines are universally available to all, CLAN's five pillars offer a clear roadmap (complete with a range of products and tools that can be shared) for those committed to redressing the inequities facing children living with CAH and other chronic health conditions in low-income settings. Our many partners have demonstrated time and again that such action is scalable, replicable and sustainable.

Communities and local champions are powerful partners in this process; they must be consulted, empowered and informing collaborative action at all times. Health professionals and health systems play a vitally important role, but it is essential for health professionals to reflect upon the fact that health alone cannot achieve health for all. Whilst the United Nations' Sustainable Development Goals (SDGs) called for global action to Leave No One Behind [96], CLAN's strategic framework for action offers a roadmap to guide collaborative action so that together we might #LeaveNoChildBehind.

Author Contributions: Conceptualization of the paper, K.A.; methodology, K.A. and P.W.; writing—original draft preparation, K.A.; writing—review and editing, A.B.Y., S.C.-C., M.E.C., C.C., V.C.D., J.H., M.I., H.N., A.P., J.R. and A.U.; supervision, P.W.; project administration, K.A., C.C.; funding acquisition, nil relevant. All authors have read and agreed to the published version of the manuscript.

Funding: This research received no external funding.

Acknowledgments: Special thanks to the many partners and stakeholders involved in the work of CLAN since 2004—it has not been possible to acknowledge all persons and organisations fully in this short paper. In Vietnam, colleagues at the National Hospital of Pediatrics in Hanoi, Children's Hospitals 1 and 2 in Ho Chi Minh City and Hue Central Hospital have played a key role, as have our Community Development Officer (CDO), Yen Thanh Mac and CAH Club Executive Members, notably Tran Trung Kien and Le. In the Philippines, Lorna R. Abad, Division of Pediatric Endocrinology, Philippine General Hospital (PGH) and Philippines Society of Pediatric Metabolism and Endocrinology (PSPME) colleagues have played an invaluable role, as have all members of CAHSAPI. In Pakistan CLAN's inaugural CDO Rabia Baloch, CLIP's Salman Munir and Yasir Naqi Khan deserve especial thanks. From Indonesia, our thanks to Muhammad Faizi and the members of KAHAKI and IKAHAK. Thank you also to Chris Cowell, Claire Henderson, Garry Warne, Jane Graham, Jim Willett, Kelly Leight, Lilea Propadalo, Lyndell Wills, Michael Moore, Michele Konheiser, Nguyen Bich Phuong, Nguyen Van Chi, Phil Koh and the late Professor Fatimah Harun, Robyn Ronai, Sue Ditchfield, and Irene Mitchelhill, as well as David, Donald and Marilyn Hansen, and Carole and Robert Armstrong for their contributions and support over many years.

Conflicts of Interest: The authors declare no conflict of interest.

Appendix A

Table A1. Examples of indicators used by CLAN (Caring & Living As Neighbours) to monitor use of knowledge to support people living with Congenital Adrenal Hyperplasia (CAH) in Vietnam.

Approach to Monitoring	Individuals & Families	Health Practitioners	Health System
Conceptual knowledge use (*changes in levels of knowledge, understanding or attitudes*)	- The CAHPepTalk tool quantitatively assesses knowledge of families - Consultation with community and health professionals to monitor needs, emerging myths and knowledge gaps, Monitoring the nature of queries received from Community in question and answer sessions at Club meetings - Co-design of Club meetings - Formal evaluation of Club meetings (written surveys; consultation)	- Number of staff attending training/educational sessions - Qualifications of staff - Number of publications - Participation in conferences/symposia - Quality of educational resources available in local language - Engagement with colleagues internationally - Requests from colleagues in other countries to replicate CLAN model	- Regular meetings and consultation with hospital executive to clarify priorities for collaborative action - Review of incidence/prevalence/mortality/health outcome data - Requests/permission given to CLAN to partner - Number of partnerships established - Use of planned action approach (Plan for CLAN) supports collaborative action - Existence/strength of national paediatric endocrinology society
Instrumental knowledge use (*changes in behavior or practice—translates into improved health outcomes*)	- height and weight recorded routinely - blood tests completed to protocol (eg 17 hydroxyprogesterone (17OHP)/renin/testosterone/androstenedione) - number of adrenal crisis admissions - mortality rates - loss to follow up - approach to sick day management/training in use of injection kits - use of alternative medicines - attendance at school - Connectivity with CAH Club members (text, phone, email, Facebook)	- Clinical guidelines established and used - Standardized approaches to inpatient and outpatient care - Participation in training (local, national and international forums) - Model replicated in Vietnam for other conditions (diabetes, osteogenesis imperfecta, Duchenne muscular dystrophy, nephrotic syndrome) - Model replicated to other countries (Philippines, Indonesia, Pakistan) - Prenatal genetic counselling and advice available	- Training of HCPs in hospitals (eg Nurse training program in Vietnam × 6 months; Health Care Professionals (HCPs) train in Australia) - Strengthen capacity of local health professionals (training, information, resources) - Newborn Screening (NBS) for CAH established - Hydrocortisone and fludrocortisone included in national register and insurance schemes - Essential testing made affordably available (17OHP, renin, genetics) - Medical education curricula strengthened

Table A1. *Cont.*

Approach to Monitoring	Individuals & Families	Health Practitioners	Health System
Strategic knowledge use (*manipulation of knowledge to attain specific power or profit goals—research as ammunition*)	- Executive members of Club working in close partnership with hospital directors, CLAN and other stakeholders on co-design of Club meetings and other initiatives - External partners engaged with Club meetings - Media/videos used to tell story - Club funding identified - Engagement with other international CAH support groups	- Patient registers established and used to monitor health outcomes and inform health system responses (e.g., need for NBS) - Publications and conference presentations raise awareness and strengthen evidence base - National Pediatric Endocrinology Society established - Involvement in regional professional networks - CAH model translated to other hospitals and countries	- RAPIA completed to inform priorities for action - Essential medicines included in World Health Organisation's Essential Medicines List for Children (WHO EMLc) - Publication and sharing of successes with other countries - Replication of successes with CAH to other chronic health conditions of childhood - Increased focus on patient and family centred care - Engagement with civil society on non-communicable diseases (NCDs) through NCD Child and IndigenousNCDs - Engagement with multilaterals - Engagement with member state governments, embassies and high commissions - Engagement with private sector

Table A2. Examples of key resources, products and tools developed by CLAN (Caring & Living As Neighbours) and available to share for the purpose of redressing inequities for children living with non-communicable diseases (NCDs).

KTA Stages	CLAN Milestone/Activities	Knowledge Creation	Products/Tools Developed
Identify the problem	International Congenital Adrenal Hyperplasia (CAH) newsletters describe situation in Vietnam Short-term humanitarian donation of essential medicines obtained for every child with CAH in Vietnam CLAN founded as Non-Government Organisation (NGO) in 2004 and incorporated as NGO with Department of Fair Trade in 2007	Access to medicine is a life-threatening problem for children living with CAH in Vietnam when essential medicines are not registered nor affordably available. National CAH Communities need to be acknowledged and supported to connect globally with one another.	CLAN constitution and policy handbook CLAN website CLAN Newsletters
Adapt knowledge to local use	Health needs assessment (HNA) conducted in Hanoi, Vietnam to learn more about challenges facing families.	Consultation with people living with CAH is essential to a comprehensive understanding of "the problem" facing families and children living with CAH in resource-poor settings	CAH HNA survey template (since translated to rheumatic heart disease (RHD), nephrotic syndrome and epilepsy)
Assess barriers to knowledge use	Analysis of responses to HNA of families, and interviews with health professionals and other stakeholders, with results published in peer-review literature. Insights informed development of CLAN's model	Power of publication of results. Development of CLAN's Strategic Framework for Action and identification of CLAN's five pillars	Publications (see references) CLAN Strategic Framework for Action
Select, tailor and implement interventions	Findings from HNA informed the development of a strategic plan to improve quality of life for every child living with CAH in Vietnam. The plan was shared with a broad range of stakeholders to promote multisectoral collaborative action and affordable/achievable/urgent actions prioritized for immediate action across the five pillars (specific examples outlined in Table A1).	Families and children must be the visual hub of all action; community development is key to sustainability. Collaboration with a broad range of multisectoral stakeholders is essential to scaling activities; communication is key to ensuring all stakeholders are aware of one another's contributions and commitments (reduces duplication and strengthens engagement. CLAN's model able to be replicated across multiple locations nationally.	Plan for CLAN—a strategic work plan, capturing activities to redress inequities according to the five pillars Successful application to the World Health Organisation's Essential Medicines List for Children (WHO EMLc) for hydrocortisone and fludrocortisone tablets Translated educational resources (booklets, books, videos, mobile phone apps etc.) Social media platforms (WhatsApp, Facebook, Twitter, Instagram)

Table A2. *Cont.*

KTA Stages	CLAN Milestone/Activities	Knowledge Creation	Products/Tools Developed
Monitor knowledge use	Evaluation of all events and activities informed a continuous quality improvement approach, and ensures priorities of people living with CAH are addressed Health outcomes were monitored by local professionals (e.g., mortality; loss to follow-up, incidence, prevalence) Close collaboration with hospital executive ensured appropriate alignment with Ministry of Health and media	Transparent and ethical project management is vital. Activities must address conceptual, instrumental and strategic knowledge use.	APPES (Asia Pacific Pediatric Endocrinology Society)—CLAN Equity (ACE) Snapshot Survey—facilitates rapid landscape analysis to identify inequities associated with paediatric endocrine conditions CLAN NGO reports: - CLAN Annual reports - CLAN reports to Australian and international governing bodies
Evaluate outcomes	RE-AIM framework informs evaluation Expansion of activities to support new Communities for CAH and other chronic conditions of childhood Support and promote professional societies and networks for health workers Development of patient registers and other systems for monitoring health outcomes, incidence and prevalence	CLAN's model is scalable and replicable across countries and health conditions. Health professionals play essential role in supporting childhood NCD communities.	CLAN Club meeting checklist CLAN Club Grant Application form Patient registers Google analytics APPES-CLAN Declaration
Sustain knowledge use	Many communities now operating independently, with own social media platforms and strategic agendas Founding of NCD Child and IndigenousNCDs facilitates broader synergies, networks and sustainability of the movement	Community development and involvement of PLW NCDs is key to sustainability of movement. There is commonality across NCDs. CLAN's work is relevant to broader NCD movement and other communities (e.g., Indigenous persons globally).	Links with individual and independent grassroots NCD communities and collaborations: - CLIP—CAH Living In Pakistan - IKAHAK and KAHAKI (CAH Communities in Indonesia) - CAHSAPI—Philippines CAH Community - FOSTEO—OI Community Indonesia International networks: - NCD Child - IndigenousNCDs

References

1. Speiser, P.W.; Arlt, W.; Auchus, R.J.; Baskin, L.S.; Conway, G.S.; Merke, D.P.; Meyer-Bahlburg, H.F.; Miller, W.L.; Murad, M.H.; Oberfield, S.E.; et al. Congenital Adrenal Hyperplasia due to steroid 21-Hydroxylase deficiency: An endocrine society clinical practice guideline. *J. Clin. Endocrinol. Metab.* **2018**, *103*, 4043–4088. [CrossRef] [PubMed]
2. Brener, A.; Segev-Becker, A.; Weintrob, N.; Stein, R.; Interator, H.; Schachter-Davidov, A.; Israeli, G.; Elkon-Tamir, E.; Lebenthal, Y.; Eyal, O.; et al. Health-related quality of life in children and adolescents with Nonclassic Congenital Adrenal Hyperplasia. *Endocr. Pract.* **2019**, *25*, 794–799. [CrossRef] [PubMed]
3. Halper, A.; Hooke, M.C.; Gonzalez-Bolanos, M.T.; Vanderburg, N.; Tran, T.N.; Torkelson, J.; Sarafoglou, K. Health-related quality of life in children with congenital adrenal hyperplasia. *Health Qual. Life Outcomes* **2017**, *15*, 194. [CrossRef] [PubMed]
4. Piane, L.D.; Rinaudo, P.; Miller, W.L. 150 Years of Congenital Adrenal Hyperplasia: Translation and Commentary of De Crecchio's Classic Paper from 1865. *Endocrinology* **2015**, *156*, 1210–1217. [CrossRef]
5. Padilla, C.D.; Therrell, B.L. Newborn screening in the Asia Pacific region. *J. Inherit. Metab. Dis.* **2007**, *30*, 490–506. [CrossRef]
6. Alfadhel, M.; Al Othaim, A.; Al Saif, S.; Al Mutairi, F.; Alsayed, M.; Rahbeeni, Z.; Alzaidan, H.; Alowain, M.; Al-Hassnan, Z.; Saeedi, M.; et al. Expanded Newborn Screening Program in Saudi Arabia: Incidence of screened disorders. *J. Paediatr. Child Health* **2017**, *53*, 585–591. [CrossRef]
7. Australian Health Ministers Advisory Council (AHMAC). CAH Condition Assessment Summary for NBS in Australia—March 2019. Available online: http://www.cancerscreening.gov.au/internet/screening/publishing.nsf/Content/C79A7D94CB73C56CCA257CEE0000EF35/$File/Congenital%20adrenal%20hyperplasia%20(CAH)%20condition%20assessment%20summary%20-%20March%202019.pdf (accessed on 30 July 2020).
8. Warne, G.L.; Armstrong, K.L.; Faunce, T.A.; Wilcken, B.; Boneh, A.; Geelhoed, E.; Craig, M.E. The case for newborn screening for congenital adrenal hyperplasia in Australia. *Med. J. Aust.* **2010**, *192*, 107. [CrossRef]
9. Gleeson, H.K.; Wiley, V.; Wilcken, B.; Elliott, E.J.; Cowell, C.; Thonsett, M.; Byrne, G.; Ambler, G. Two-year pilot study of newborn screening for congenital adrenal hyperlasia in New South Wales compared with nationwide case surveillance in Australia. *J. Paediatr. Child Health* **2008**, *44*, 554–559. [CrossRef]
10. Wu, J.Y.; Sudeep; Cowley, D.M.; Harris, M.; McGown, I.N.; Cotterill, A.M. Is it time to commence newborn screening for congenital adrenal hyperplasia in Australia? *Med. J. Aust.* **2011**, *195*, 260–262. [CrossRef]
11. CAHSGA (Congenital Adrenal Hyperplasia Support Group Australia) Incorporated. Available online: http://www.cah.org.au (accessed on 30 July 2020).
12. CARES Foundation. Available online: https://caresfoundation.org (accessed on 30 July 2020).
13. CLAN (Caring & Living As Neighbours) Incorporated. Available online: www.clanchildhealth.org (accessed on 30 July 2020).
14. Armstrong, K.; Henderson, C.; Hoan, N.; Warne, G.L. Living with Congenital Adrenal Hyperplasia in Vietnam: A Survey of Parents. *J. Pediatr. Endocrinol. Metab.* **2006**, *19*, 1207–1224. [CrossRef]
15. Armstrong, K.L. Working together so we #LeaveNoChildBehind. In Proceedings of the 9th Biennial Scientific Meeting of APPES (Asia Pacific Pediatric Endocrinology Society), Tokyo, Japan, 17–20 November 2016.
16. Roe, M.T.; Mahaffey, K.W.; Ezekowitz, J.A.; Alexander, J.H.; Goodman, S.G.; Hernandez, A.F.; Temple, T.; Berdan, L.; Califf, R.M.; Harrington, R.A.; et al. The future of cardiovascular clinical research in North America and beyond—Addressing challenges and leveraging opportunities through unique academic and grassroots collaborations. *Am. Heart J.* **2015**, *169*, 743–750. [CrossRef] [PubMed]
17. Armstrong, K.L.; Nguyen, H.T.; Nguyen, L.T.; Le, V.H.; Thoai, L.H.; Binh, T.; Hoang, T.T.D.; Mac, Y.T.; Tong, A.; Hodson, E. Understanding the challenges facing children and families living with Nephrotic Syndrome in Vietnam: A survey of families. In *Pediatric Nephrology*; Springer: New York, NY, USA, 2013.
18. Merriam, S.B.; Johnson-Bailey, J.; Lee, M.-Y.; Kee, Y.; Ntseane, G.; Muhamad, M. Power and positionality: Negotiating insider/outsider status within and across cultures. *Int. J. Lifelong Educ.* **2001**, *20*, 405–416. [CrossRef]
19. Ozano, K.; Khatri, R. Reflexivity, positionality and power in cross-cultural participatory action research with research assistants in rural Cambodia. *Educ. Action Res.* **2017**, *26*, 190–204. [CrossRef]
20. Bhaskar, R. *A Realist Theory of Science*; Taylor and Francis Group, Routledge: London, UK; New York, NY, USA, 1978.

21. Easton, G. Critical realism in case study research. *Ind. Mark. Manag.* **2010**, *39*, 118–128. [CrossRef]
22. Fletcher, A.J. Applying critical realism in qualitative research: Methodology meets method. *Int. J. Soc. Res. Methodol.* **2016**, *20*, 181–194. [CrossRef]
23. McEvoy, P.; Richards, D.A. A critical realist rationale for using a combination of quantitative and qualitative methods. *J. Res. Nurs.* **2006**, *11*, 66–78. [CrossRef]
24. Baum, F.; MacDougall, C.; Smith, D. Participatory action research. *J. Epidemiol. Community Health* **2006**, *60*, 854–857. [CrossRef]
25. NCD Alliance—"Our Views, Our Voices". Available online: https://ncdalliance.org/what-we-do/capacity-development/our-views-our-voices (accessed on 27 August 2020).
26. Harrison, H.; Birks, M.; Franklin, R.; Mills, J. Case Study Research: Foundations and Methodological Orientations. *Forum Qual. Soc. Res.* **2017**, *18*. [CrossRef]
27. Graham, I.D.; Logan, J.; Harrison, M.B.; Straus, S.E.; Tetroe, J.; Caswell, W.; Robinson, N. Lost in knowledge translation: Time for a map? *J. Contin. Educ. Health Prof.* **2006**, *26*, 13–24. [CrossRef]
28. World Health Organisation (WHO)—Knowledge-to-Action (KTA) Framework. Available online: https://www.who.int/reproductivehealth/topics/best_practices/greatproject_KTAframework/en/ (accessed on 30 July 2020).
29. Yin, R. *Case Study Research: Design and Methods*, 5th ed.; Sage Publications: Thousand Oaks, CA, USA, 2014.
30. Warne, G. The state of children and teenagers with CAH in Vietnam. In *CARES Foundation Fall Newsletter*; CARES Foundation: Union, NJ, USA, 2004; p. 12.
31. Konheiser, M. *My Vietnam Experience, in CARES Foundation Fall Newsletter*; CARES Foundation: Union, NJ, USA, 2004; pp. 10–11.
32. Australian Government, Department of Health—Medicare. Available online: https://www.health.gov.au/health-topics/medicare (accessed on 30 July 2020).
33. Mylan Australia. Available online: https://www.mylan.com.au (accessed on 30 July 2020).
34. Bristol Myers Squibb. Available online: https://www.bms.com/about-us/our-company/new-bristol-myers-squibb.html (accessed on 30 July 2020).
35. CLAN (Caring & Living As Neighbours) Annual Report 2005. Available online: https://www.clanchildhealth.org/uploads/8/3/3/6/83366650/clan_2005_annual_report.pdf (accessed on 30 August 2020).
36. CLAN (Caring & Living As Neighbours) Annual Report 2006. Available online: https://www.clanchildhealth.org/uploads/8/3/3/6/83366650/clan_2006_-_annual_report.pdf (accessed on 30 August 2020).
37. CLAN (Caring & Living As Neighbours) Annual Report 2007. Available online: https://www.clanchildhealth.org/uploads/8/3/3/6/83366650/clan_2007_annual_report.pdf (accessed on 30 August 2020).
38. Consensus Statement on 21-Hydroxylase Deficiency from The European Society for Paediatric Endocrinology and The Lawson Wilkins Pediatric Endocrine Society. *Horm. Res. Paediatr.* **2002**, *58*, 188–195. [CrossRef]
39. CLAN (Caring & Living As Neighbours) Annual Report 2008. Available online: https://www.clanchildhealth.org/uploads/8/3/3/6/83366650/2008-clan-annual-report.pdf (accessed on 30 August 2020).
40. Hsu, C.Y.; Rivkees, S.A. *Congenital Adrenal Hyperplasia: A Parent's Guide*; AuthorHouse: Bloomington, IN, USA, 2005; p. 290.
41. Hsu, C.Y.; Rivkees, S.A. *Tăng Sản thượng thận Bẩm Sinh*; Nhà Xuất Bản Y Học.: Hanoi, Vietnam, 2011; p. 323.
42. CLAN (Caring & Living As Neighbours) Annual Report 2011–2012. Available online: https://www.clanchildhealth.org/uploads/8/3/3/6/83366650/fy10-11_clan_annual_report_[email]-1.pdf (accessed on 30 August 2020).
43. Sayer, A. *Realism and Social Science*; Sage: London, UK, 2000.
44. Serrat, O. The Five Whys Technique. 2009. Available online: https://www.adb.org/sites/default/files/publication/27641/five-whys-technique.pdf (accessed on 30 July 2020).
45. Marmot, M. Social determinants of health inequalities. *Lancet* **2005**, *365*, 1099–1104. [CrossRef]
46. World Health Organization. *World Health Organisation Model List of Essential Medicines for Children*, 7th ed.; World Health Organization: Geneva, Switzerland, 2019.
47. ACFID (Australian Council For International Development). Available online: https://acfid.asn.au (accessed on 30 August 2020).
48. International Insulin Foundation (IIF) Project in Vietnam. Available online: http://www.access2insulin.org/iifs-project-in-vietnam.html (accessed on 30 July 2020).
49. CLAN (Caring & Living As Neighbours). *Child-Friendly CAH Rights Flyer*; CLAN Inc.: Sydney, Australia, 2017. Available online: https://www.clanchildhealth.org/cah.html (accessed on 30 August 2020).

50. VIDEO—July 2012 CAH Club Hanoi, Vietnam. Available online: https://www.youtube.com/watch?v=QcynUyhzhV4 (accessed on 30 August 2020).
51. APPES. The Tokyo Declaration of the 9th Biennial Scientific Meeting of the Asia Pacific Pediatric Endocrinology Society (APPES). In Proceedings of the APPES Conference, Tokyo, Japan, 17–20 November 2016.
52. Zainuddin, A.A.; Grover, S.R.; Shamsuddin, K.; Mahdy, Z.A. Research on Quality of Life in Female Patients with Congenital Adrenal Hyperplasia and Issues in Developing Nations. *J. Pediatric Adolesc. Gynaecol.* **2013**, *26*, 296–304. [CrossRef]
53. Mitchelhill, I.; Armstrong, K.; Craig, M.; Dung, V.C.; Thao, B.P.; Khanh, N.N.; Ngoc, T.B.; Hoang, T.T.D.; Quynh, H.; Tran, D.T.P.; et al. Evaluation of parental knowledge after establishing CAH clubs in Vietnam & Indonesia. *Int. J. Pediatric Endocrinol.* **2015**, *2015* (Suppl. 1), P53.
54. APPES (Asia Pacific Pediatric Endocrinology Society). Available online: https://www.appes.org (accessed on 30 July 2020).
55. CLAN (Caring & Living As Neighbours) Annual Report 2016–2017. Available online: https://www.clanchildhealth.org/uploads/8/3/3/6/83366650/clan_2016-2017_annual_report__1_.pdf (accessed on 30 August 2020).
56. Glasgow, R.E.; Vogt, T.M.; Boles, S.M. Evaluating the public health impact of health promotion interventions: The RE-AIM framework. *Am. J. Public Health* **1999**, *89*, 1322–1327. [CrossRef]
57. Dung, V.C.; Thao, B.P.; Ngoc, C.T.B.; Khanh, N.N.; Dat, N.P.; Hoan, N.T.; Mai, D.T.; Craig, M. Updated registry of congenital adrenal hyperplasia at the north pediatric referral centre of Vietnam. *Int. J. Pediatr. Endocrinol.* **2015**, *2015*, P49. [CrossRef]
58. Huynh, Q.T.; Thuy, H.; Armstrong, K.; Craig, M. Effectiveness of diabetes and congenital adrenal hyperplasia meeting clubs. *Int. J. Pediatr. Endocrinol.* **2013**, *2013*, P134. [CrossRef]
59. Ngoc, C.T.B.; Dung, V.C.; Thao, B.P.; Khanh, N.N.; Dat, N.P.; Craig, M.; Ellard, S.; Hoan, N.T. Phenotype, genotype of neonatal diabetes mellitus due to insulin gene mutation. *Int. J. Pediatr. Endocrinol.* **2015**, *2015*, P12. [CrossRef]
60. Can, T.B.N.; Dung, V.C.; Bui, T.P.; Nguyen, K.N.; Flanagan, S.E.; Ellard, S.; Craig, M.; Nguyen, D.P.; Nguyen, H.T. Neonatal diabetes mellitus: Genotype, phenotype and outcome. *Ann. Transl. Med.* **2015**. [CrossRef]
61. Can, T.B.N.; Dung, V.C.; Thao, B.P.; Khanh, N.N.; Dat, N.P.; Sian, E.; Thi, H.N. The Result of Sulphonylureas Treatment in Patients with Neonatal Diabetes Mellitus due to kcnj11/abcc8 Gene Mutations in Vietnam. In Proceedings of the ESPE Dublin (European Society for Paediatric Endocrinology Conference), Hormone Research in Paediatrics (82), Dublin, Ireland, 18–22 September 2014.
62. Chi, D.V.; Tran, T.H.; Nguyen, D.H.; Luong, L.H.; Le, P.T.; Ta, M.H.; Ngo, H.T.T.; Nguyen, M.P.; Le-Anh, T.P.; Nguyen, D.P.; et al. Novel variants of CYP21A2 in Vietnamese patients with congenital adrenal hyperplasia. *Mol. Genet. Genom. Med.* **2019**, *7*, e623. [CrossRef]
63. Chi, D.V. (National Hospital of Pediatrics, Hanoi, Vietnam). Personal communication, 2020.
64. Chi, D.V.; Nguyen, N.L.; Nguyen, H.H.; Nguyen, T.K.L.; Tran, T.H.; Ta, T.V.; Tran, V.K. A novel nonsense mutation in the CYP21A2 gene of a Vietnamese patient with congenital adrenal hyperplasia. In Proceedings of the Biomedical Research and Therapy—Abstract Proceeding: International Conference "Innovations in Cancer Research and Regenerative Medicine 2017", Ho Chi Minh City, Vietnam, 10–13 September 2017.
65. Armstrong, K.L.; Ditchfield, S.; Henderson, C.; Nguyen, H.T.; Bui, T.P.; Warne, G. Young people living with CAH in Vietnam: A survivor's cohort (Poster presentation). In Proceedings of the 2008 State Population Health Conference: Public Health Research for the Real World, Hindmarsh, South Australia, 18 October 2008.
66. Varni, J.W. The PedsQL TM Measurement Model for the Pediatric Quality of Life Inventory. Available online: https://www.pedsql.org/index.html (accessed on 20 September 2020).
67. CLAN (Caring & Living As Neighbours), VIDEO—Happy and Healthy with CAH. 2012. Available online: https://www.youtube.com/watch?v=83b05k7MGQ4 (accessed on 30 August 2020).
68. Proceedings of the the Second Meeting of the Subcommittee of the Expert Committee on the Selection and Use of Essential Medicines, Geneva, Switzerland, 29 September–3 October 2008. Available online: https://www.who.int/selection_medicines/committees/subcommittee/2/Fludrocortisone_MAIN.pdf (accessed on 30 August 2020).
69. Facebook Group for CAHSAPI (the Philippines CAH Support Group). Available online: https://www.facebook.com/groups/170268589670584 (accessed on 30 July 2020).

70. Republic of the Philippines Department of Health, Newborn Screening Program. Available online: https://www.doh.gov.ph/newborn-screening (accessed on 10 August 2020).
71. Utari, A.; Ariani, M.D.; Ediati, A.; Juniarto, A.Z.; Faradz, S.M.H. Mortality Problems of Congenital Adrenal Hyperplasia in Central Java-Indonesia: 12 years experiences. In Proceedings of the 9th Biannual Meeting of the Asia Pacific Pediatric Endocrine Society (APPES)—50th Scientific Meeting of Japanese Society for Pediatric Endocrinology (JSPE), Tokyo, Japan, 16–20 November 2016.
72. VIDEO—Tatap Masa Depan dengan Optimis—Look to the Future with Optimism. A CAH Resource for Families in Bahasa Indonesia. Available online: https://m.youtube.com/watch?index=3&list=UUOYPyehX3HOgmluHNFEP00A&t=0s&v=Rt7kaTQDrSQ#menu (accessed on 30 August 2020).
73. Utari, A.; Ediati, A. Bacaan Untuk Remaja Putri Dengan Hiperplasia Adrenal Kongenital—Readings for Young Women with Congenital Adrenal Hyperplasia. Available online: https://www.clanchildhealth.org/uploads/8/3/3/6/83366650/cah_book_for_adolescent_girls_bahasa_indonesia.pdf (accessed on 30 August 2020).
74. Warne, G.; Sung, V.; Raza, S.R.; Khan, Y.N.; Armstrong, K.L. Application for inclusion of Hydrocortisone tablets in the WHO Model List of Essential Medicines for Children. In Proceedings of the the Expert Committee on the Selection and Use of Essential Medicines, Children's Essential Medicines List, World Health Organization, Geneva, Switzerland, 29 September–3 October 2008.
75. Warne, G.; Raza, S.R.; Khan, Y.N.; Armstrong, K.L. Application for inclusion of Fludrocortisone tablets in the WHO Model List of Essential Medicines for Children. In Proceedings of the the Second Meeting of the Subcommittee of the Expert Committee on the Selection and Use of Essential Medicines, Geneva, Switzerland, 29 September–3 October 2008.
76. SPED. Society of Paediatric Endocrinology and Diabetes—Pakistan. Available online: http://sped.org.pk (accessed on 30 August 2020).
77. Pfizer Australia. Available online: https://www.pfizer.com.au (accessed on 27 August 2020).
78. CLAN Inc. Video: Working together for the CAH Community in Pakistan (CLAN and NICH), November 2016. Available online: https://www.youtube.com/watch?v=begn3hQ6pNg&index=8&list=UUOYPyehX3HOgmluHNFEP00A&t=0s (accessed on 30 August 2020).
79. World Health Organisation. World Health Organisation Constitution (adopted by the International Health Conference in New York, USA on 22 July 1946, and Came into Force on 7 April 1948). Available online: https://apps.who.int/gb/bd/PDF/bd47/EN/constitution-en.pdf?ua=1 (accessed on 30 August 2020).
80. United Nations Convention on the Rights of the Child. Adopted and Opened for Signature, Ratification and Accession by General Assembly Resolution 44/25 of 20 November 1989, with Entry into Force 2 September 1990 in Accordance with Article 49. Available online: https://www.ohchr.org/en/professionalinterest/pages/crc.aspx (accessed on 30 August 2020).
81. Wishbone Day. Available online: http://www.wishboneday.com/p/about.html (accessed on 30 August 2020).
82. NCD Child. Available online: http://www.ncdchild.org (accessed on 30 August 2020).
83. United Nations General Assembly. Political Declaration of the High-level Meeting of the General Assembly on the Prevention and Control of Non-Communicable Diseases. In proceedings of the 66th session (agenda item 117) of the United Nations General Assembly in 2011. Available online: https://www.who.int/nmh/events/un_ncd_summit2011/political_declaration_en.pdf?ua (accessed on 30 August 2020).
84. World Health Organisation. *Omnibus Resolution—Follow-Up to the Political Declaration of the High-Level Meeting of the General Assembly on the Prevention and Control of Non-communicable Diseases*; Agenda item 13.1 and 13.2; WHA66.10.; World Health Organisation: Geneva, Switzerland, 2013.
85. IndigenousNCDs. Available online: www.indigenousncds.org (accessed on 30 July 2020).
86. Bukhman, G.; Mocumbi, A.O.; Atun, R.; Becker, A.E.; Bhutta, Z.; Binagwaho, A.; Clinton, C.; Coates, M.M.; Dain, K.; Ezzati, M.; et al. The Lancet NCDI Poverty Commission: Bridging a gap in universal health coverage for the poorest billion. *Lancet* **2020**. [CrossRef]
87. Maslow, A.H. A theory of human motivation. *Psychol. Rev.* **1943**, *50*, 370–396. [CrossRef]
88. World Health Organisation. WHO Launches First-Ever Insulin Prequalification Programme to Expand Access to Life-Saving Treatment for Diabetes. Available online: https://www.who.int/news-room/detail/13-11-2019-who-launches-first-ever-insulin-prequalification-programme-to-expand-access-to-life-saving-treatment-for-diabetes (accessed on 27 August 2020).

89. Finlay, S.M.; Armstrong, K.L. Indigenous languages must play a role in tackling noncommunicable diseases. In *2019 BMJ Collection "Solutions for Non-Communicable Disease Prevention and Control"*. Available online: https://www.bmj.com/NCD-solutions (accessed on 30 August 2020).
90. Utari, A.; Ediati, A.; Dhaliwal, R.; Freeman, J.; Armstrong, K. Girl power! How a novel booklet developed to provide psychological support for teenage girls living with CAH in Indonesia is helping to redress health inequities regionally in Poster. In Proceedings of the (P02.18) at the November 2018 APPES (Asia Pacific Pediatric Endocrinology Society) Conference, Chiang Mai, Thailand, 7–10 November 2018.
91. United Nations Sustainable Development Goals (SDGs). Available online: https://www.un.org/sustainabledevelopment/sustainable-development-goals/ (accessed on 27 August 2020).
92. Rodgers, R. *Do-Re-Mi, in The Sound of Music*; Rodgers and Hammerstein: New York, NY, USA, 1959.
93. Kluge, H.H.P.; Wickramasinghe, K.; Rippin, H.L.; Mendes, R.; Peters, D.H.; Kontsevaya, A.; Breda, J. Prevention and control of non-communicable diseases in the COVID-19 response. *Lancet* **2020**, *395*, 1678–1680. [CrossRef]
94. World Bank. Profiles of the New Poor Due to the COVID-19 Pandemic. Available online: https://www.worldbank.org/en/topic/poverty/brief/Profiles-of-the-new-poor-due-to-the-COVID-19-pandemic (accessed on 30 August 2020).
95. World Health Organisation. COVAX: Working for Global Equitable Access to COVID-19 Vaccines. Available online: https://www.who.int/initiatives/act-accelerator/covax (accessed on 21 September 2020).
96. United Nations, The Sustainable Development Goals Report. 2016. Available online: https://unstats.un.org/sdgs/report/2016/leaving-no-one-behind (accessed on 30 August 2020).

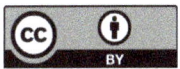

© 2020 by the authors. Licensee MDPI, Basel, Switzerland. This article is an open access article distributed under the terms and conditions of the Creative Commons Attribution (CC BY) license (http://creativecommons.org/licenses/by/4.0/).

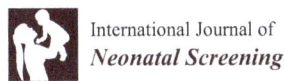

International Journal of
Neonatal Screening

Article

Update on the Swedish Newborn Screening for Congenital Adrenal Hyperplasia Due to 21-Hydroxylase Deficiency

Rolf H. Zetterström [1,2], Leif Karlsson [1,3], Henrik Falhammar [2,4], Svetlana Lajic [3,5] and Anna Nordenström [1,3,5,*]

1. Centre for Inherited Metabolic Diseases, Karolinska University Hospital, SE-171 76 Stockholm, Sweden; rolf.zetterstrom@sll.se (R.H.Z.); leif.karlsson@sll.se (L.K.)
2. Department of Molecular Medicine and Surgery, Karolinska Institutet, SE-171 76 Stockholm, Sweden; henrik.falhammar@ki.se
3. Department of Women's and Children's Health, Karolinska Institutet, SE-171 76 Stockholm, Sweden; svetlana.lajic@ki.se
4. Department of Endocrinology, Metabolism and Diabetes, Karolinska University Hospital, SE-171 77 Stockholm, Sweden
5. Pediatric Endocrinology Unit, Astrid Lindgren´s Children's Hospital, Karolinska University Hospital, SE-171 76 Stockholm, Sweden
* Correspondence: anna.nordenstrom@ki.se

Received: 11 August 2020; Accepted: 26 August 2020; Published: 28 August 2020

Abstract: Congenital adrenal hyperplasia (CAH) was the fourth disorder added to the national Swedish neonatal screening program in 1986, and approximately 115,000 newborns are screened annually. Dried blood spot (DBS) screening with measurement of 17-hydroxyprogesterone (17OHP) is also offered to older children moving to Sweden from countries lacking a national DBS screening program. Here, we report an update on the CAH screening from January 2011 until December 2019. *Results*: During the study period, 1,030,409 newborns and 34,713 older children were screened. In total, 87 newborns were verified to have CAH, which gives an overall positive predictive value (PPV) of 11% and 21% for term infants. Including the five missed CAH cases identified during this period, this gives an incidence of 1:11,200 of CAH in Sweden. Among the older children, 12 of 14 recalled cases were found to be true positive for CAH. All patients were genotyped as part of the clinical follow-up and 70% of the newborns had salt wasting (SW) CAH and 92% had classic CAH (i.e., SW and simple virilizing (SV) CAH). In the group of 12 older children, none had SW CAH and two had SV CAH. *Conclusion*: The incidence of classic CAH is relatively high in Sweden. Early genetic confirmation with *CYP21A2* genotyping has been a valuable complement to the analysis of 17OHP to predict disease severity, make treatment decisions and for the follow-up and evaluation of the screening program.

Keywords: neonatal screening; congenital adrenal hyperplasia; CAH; 21-hydroxylase deficiency; *CYP21A2*; dried blood spots; DBS; positive predictive value; PPV

1. Introduction

Congenital adrenal hyperplasia (CAH) is in more than 95% of cases due to 21-hydroxylase deficiency (21OHD) caused by mutations in the *CYP21A2* gene [1,2]. It results in varying degrees of cortisol and aldosterone deficiency and at the same time an overproduction of androgens. If untreated, severe forms lead to lethal adrenal crisis in the neonatal period. Before neonatal screening, there was often a preponderance of females among patients with CAH since girls were more often identified at birth due to the prenatal virilization of external genitalia [3,4].

Measurements of 17-hydroxyprogesterone (17OHP), the metabolite before the enzymatic block, have been used as a marker for the disease [5]. Neonatal screening using filter paper cards was first accomplished in the 1970s [6]. However, neonatal screening for CAH has a relatively high false positive rate, which may have delayed its general implementation [7]. Gestational age and/or birth weight related cut-off levels have been used to try to solve this problem [8–11]. Second tier strategies using tandem mass spectrometry measuring additional steroid metabolites and using ratios of metabolites are also used and have been shown to be useful in reducing the number of false positive cases [7,12,13]. During the past decade, neonatal screening has been implemented in an increasing number of countries over the world [1].

The molecular genetics for CAH is well described [14,15]. There is a limited number of mutations, including deletion of the entire *CYP21A2* gene, that make up more than 90% of the alleles described in patients worldwide. The genotype and phenotype correlation is good, making it possible to predict the clinical severity of the disease.

Neonatal screening for CAH started in Sweden in 1986 [16]. Since then, more than 3.5 million babies have been screened. There is one national screening laboratory in Sweden managing more than 100,000 samples per year. Newborn screening is not mandatory in Sweden, but more than 99.5% of all newborns are screened. The results of the screening program between 1986 and 2011 have been reported previously [17]. Here, we extend the reporting period to also include newborns screened until 2019 and we also include the results from screening older children moving to Sweden who had not been screened for CAH in the neonatal period.

2. Materials and Methods

The dried blood spot (DBS) samples were collected as soon as possible after 48 h after birth (48–72 h) on Perkin Elmer 226 Ahlstrom paper (Perkin Elmer, Waltham, MA, USA). The families were given written and oral information at the time of sampling and an opt out procedure was employed. DBS screening was also offered to older children, below the age of 9 years, that moved to Sweden from countries lacking a national newborn screening program for CAH.

The 17OHP was measured using GSP® instruments (Perkin Elmer, Turku, Finland). Between 2011 and 2014, AutoDELFIA® was used (Perkin Elmer, Turku, Finland). Gestational age (GA) related cut-off levels were used and the cut-off level for term infants born after GA 37 weeks was 60 nmol/L in plasma and assuming a hematocrit of 50% in the blood samples. For infants born at GA 35–36, the cut-off level was 100 nmol/L, and for preterm babies born before GA 35 weeks, the cut-off level was 350 nmol/L. Children below the age of 9 years moving to Sweden were also recommended DBS screening, according to the instructions by the Swedish Board of Health and Welfare, if not screened as newborns. The cut-off level for these children was set to 50 nmol/L.

All cases with a 17OHP above the cut-off level were considered positive at the screening test and recalled for a clinical review. A case was considered true positive when diagnostic tests analyzed locally and a second DBS sample were evaluated together with the clinical assessment of the child and the diagnosis was clear. All diagnosed patients and cases with a suspected or uncertain diagnosis were genotyped for confirmation of diagnosis. Samples collected prior to 48 h of age were also analyzed when the diagnosis was suspected clinically due to virilization of the external genitalia or family history of CAH.

Genotyping was performed in one laboratory in Sweden, at the Department of Clinical Genetics, the Karolinska University Hospital in Stockholm. The whole *CYP21A2* gene was sequenced using Sanger sequencing.

The patients were clustered into genotype groups based on the severity of the milder allele. Generally, null and I2 splice, genotype groups A and B, respectively, are associated with the salt wasting (SW) phenotype. I172N is associated with SV CAH (group C), and V281L with non-classic (NC) CAH (group E). P30L results in a phenotype between SV and NC and was here defined as group D.

The study was approved by the Swedish Ethical Review Authority (approval 18 December 2019, number 2019-05816).

3. Results

The results from the first of January 2011 until the 31 December 2019 are reported. A total of 1,030,409 million newborn babies and 34,713 children below the age of 9 years and who had moved to Sweden were screened during this period. A summary of recalls, true positive and false negative cases are shown in Table 1. Among 791 recalled newborn babies, 87 were identified to have CAH. In Figure 1A, the percentage of recalls in the different age groups is shown.

Table 1. All recalls, true positive cases, false negative cases and PPV values for the CAH screening in Sweden of more than one million children between 2011 and 2019.

Age Group	Total Recalls	True Positive Cases	False Negative Cases	PPV
GA < 35 w	214	0	2	-
GA 35–36 w	189	4	2	2%
Term	388	83	1	22%
Total newborns	791	87	5	11%
Older children	14	12	-	86%

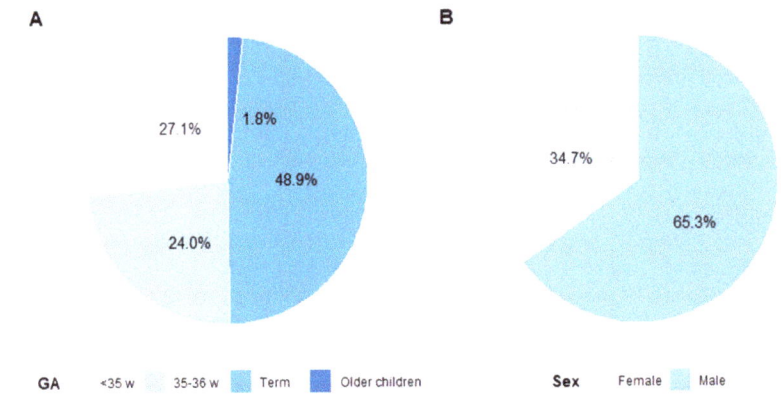

Figure 1. Gestational age (**A**) and sex (**B**) distribution of all recalls in the neonatal screening program for CAH in Sweden during the study period.

The incidence of 21OHD in newborn babies was 1:11,200 and 92% of the detected cases had the classic form of CAH (SW and SV forms); 70% of the newborns were found to have SW CAH. The incidence of classic CAH was 1:12,300 and the NC form 1:79,300. Including the P30L in the NC genotype group gave an incidence of 1:54,200. In the group of older children, none had SW CAH, as could be expected (see below). Almost half, 48.9%, of the recalled children were born at term ≥37 weeks and 51.1% were preterm, born in or before GW 36. Older children screened when moving to Sweden represented 1.8% of recalls.

The positive predictive value (PPV) for newborns was overall 11%. For term babies, the PPV was 21%, and for preterm infants, the PPV was 1%. The false positive rate overall was 0.068%, and the false negative rate was 5.4%. The overall sensitivity was 94.6% and the specificity was 99.9%.

During the study period, more males than females were identified: 49 males and 38 females (see Figure 1B). Sixty-five percent of recalls and 56% of true positives were males. For all patients, *CYP21A2* genotyping was performed. Mutations were identified in all but one of the patients. He had markedly elevated 17OHP, >670 nmol/L in the screening, and extensive steroid hormone investigations indicated 21OHD but genetic investigations failed to identify a genetic diagnosis of adrenal enzyme deficiency thus far. The number of patients in each genotype group is shown in Figure 2A. The level of 17OHP in the screening sample versus the genotype group is shown in Figure 2B.

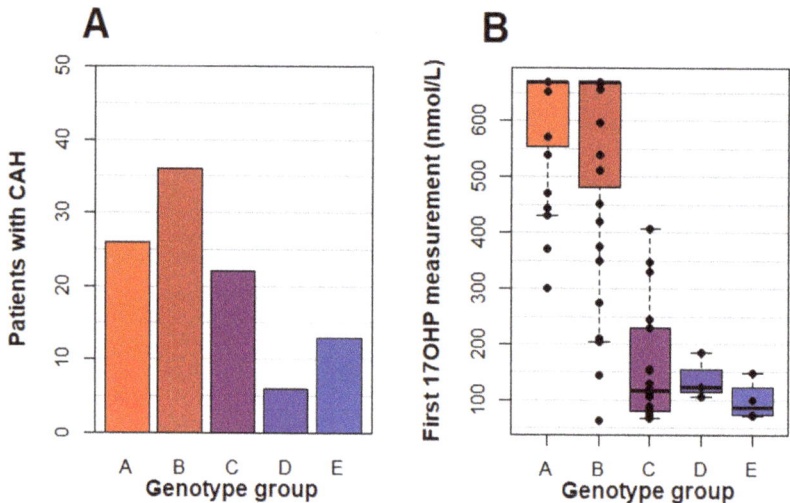

Figure 2. Distribution of all CAH patients' *CYP21A2* genotype groups (n = 103) (**A**) and correlations of the 17OHP values in the neonatal screening samples to the *CYP21A2* genotype groups (**B**). The 17OHP level is given up to 670 nmol/L by the laboratory, which means that higher levels are reported as >670 nmol/L. Five patients are not included in graph B due to a missing genotype in one case, missing 17OHP in one case and sampling prior to 48 h in three cases.

During the 9-year study period, five CAH patients were identified to have been missed by the screening program; see Table 1. One female (GW 34 with the I2 splice genotype (group B)) had a 17OHP value of 200 nmol/L, one female with SV CAH (GW 39) had 17OHP 39 nmol/L, one female with the P30L genotype (group D) (GW 36) had 17OHP 61 nmol/L, and two individuals with NC CAH (male GW 33 and female GW 35) had 17OHP values of 44 and 51 nmol/L, respectively.

In total, 14 children with an age between 13 months and 8 years were recalled. Twelve of these children were found to have CAH; see Table 1. Two had SV CAH, two had the P30L genotype (group D), and eight had NC CAH. In two cases, the 17OHP value normalized in the follow-up; in one child, a specific diagnosis was not identified, and in the other case, the elevated 17OHP was thought to be due to stress and malnutrition when the first sample was taken.

4. Discussion

This is an update on the neonatal screening for CAH in Sweden, from January 2011 until December 2019. During this period, a little more than one million newborn babies and almost 35,000 older children that moved into Sweden were screened. The majority (92%) of the patients identified in the screening had the classic form of the disease. The overall incidence of CAH in newborns in Sweden, 1:11,200, was somewhat higher than in many other countries, despite a lower incidence of NC CAH [3]. The incidence of classic CAH was 1:12,300 and of NC CAH 1:54,300.

Children moving to Sweden from countries without neonatal screening were offered screening up to the age of 8 years. Among these 35,000 children, the incidence was considerably higher, 1:2900. Two patients had the classic SV form of CAH and would definitely have benefited from earlier diagnosis. The others belonged to the genotype groups P30L and NC CAH, with no risk of salt-losing crisis [18]. The overall aim of the screening is to prevent neonatal salt-losing crises and death. However, our impression is that some of the children with NC CAH benefit from being detected early. Treatment with hydrocortisone has only been initiated if they had clinical symptoms, markedly accelerated bone age or a stimulated cortisol level that was considered insufficient for age. In some cases, the families were advised to give stress doses of hydrocortisone in case of fever without starting regular treatment. It is known that some individuals with the NC genotype develop more symptoms and have an insufficient maximum capacity to produce cortisol compared to others, despite the same *CYP21A2* genotype (18). In our experience, the children with NC CAH identified in the neonatal screening did not seldom require treatment, suggesting that being identified in the neonatal screening is an indication that they have a genetic background that predisposes them to produce more adrenal androgens and hence develop symptoms.

The efficiency of the screening program depends on the samples being collected early enough to avoid salt-losing crisis [17]. The earlier time of sampling, from 72 to 120 h to as soon as possible after 48 h, implemented prior to the extension of the Swedish national screening program in 2010, was therefore positive also for the screening for CAH. The turnaround time and the feedback to the health professionals regarding an elevated sample are all important steps for an efficient screening program (see review article in this issue).

The earlier time of sampling may have affected the distribution of males and females, with 65% of recalls and 56% of true positives being males. In our previous study, the males constituted 61.5% and females 38.5% of recalls but the number of true positive cases was similar between males and females [17]. The PPV was somewhat lower in boys than in girls. Interestingly, four of the missed cases were females, indicating a somewhat lower overall sensitivity for females or, more likely, the girls were more often identified clinically due to signs of increased androgen production when they sought medical attention. However, there was no significant sex difference in the sensitivity, with 87.2% for boys and 81.6% for the girls, despite a PPV for boys of 11% and for girls of 17%, as we previously reported [17].

The aim of the newborn screening for CAH is to avoid salt-losing crisis and neonatal death. The false negative cases among infants born full-term have most often had less severe forms of CAH, the I172N and the V281L genotype groups, with low or no risk of developing neonatal salt-losing crisis. Over the years, four patients in the I2 splice genotype group have been missed by the screening, three reported previously [17]. They were diagnosed later during childhood but none of them had developed any adrenal crisis. The one reported here, however, had an uncertain gestational age and other medical issues requiring intervention. It is known that the genotype and phenotype correlation is especially difficult for individuals in the I2 splice genotype group. A few patients with this genotype have been reported not to develop salt crises and there are individuals who were identified when investigated as presumed carriers but never developed any symptoms of cortisol deficiency or increased adrenal androgen production [3,19].

Further improvement in screening efficiency and outcome will require implementation of a second tier. Between September 2011 and May 2013, we performed second tier tandem mass spectrometry analysis on term children with 17OHP values between 60 and 100 nmol/L, measuring 17OHP, androstenedione, cortisol, 21-deoxycortisol and 11-deoxycortisol [20]. Work is now in progress to implement MS/MS second tier testing as a routine procedure and to start using the Collaborative Laboratory Integrated Reports (see www.clir.mayo.edu and Special Issue in this journal).

5. Conclusions

The newborn screening for CAH in Sweden had an incidence of 1:11,200 and the present overall PPV was 11% and for full term infants was 21%. Screening of older children moving to Sweden from countries lacking DBS screening for CAH has also proven to be valuable. All infants identified were genotyped, which enabled classification of the disease severity. This lends valuable support in clinical decision-making concerning treatment and facilitates assessment of the efficacy of the screening program.

Author Contributions: Conceptualization, methodology, formal analysis and investigation, R.H.Z., L.K., H.F., S.L. and A.N.; writing—review and editing, R.H.Z., L.K., H.F., S.L. and A.N. All authors have read and agreed to the published version of the manuscript.

Funding: This was funded by Stockholm County Council and Karolinska Institutet (ALF-SLL) 108223.

Acknowledgments: All staff of the PKU laboratory is acknowledged for skillful performance.

Conflicts of Interest: The authors declare no conflict of interest.

Abbreviations

CAH	Congenital adrenal hyperplasia
21OHD	21-hydroxylase deficiency
17OHP	17-hydroxyprogesterone
SW	Salt wasting
SV	Simple virilizing
NC	Non-classic
GA	Gestational age
PPV	Positive predictive value
DBS	Dried blood spot

References

1. Speiser, P.W.; Arlt, W.; Auchus, R.J.; Baskin, L.S.; Conway, G.S.; Merke, D.P.; Meyer-Bahlburg, H.F.L.; Miller, W.L.; Murad, M.H.; Oberfield, S.E.; et al. Congenital Adrenal Hyperplasia Due to Steroid 21-Hydroxylase Deficiency: An Endocrine Society Clinical Practice Guideline. *J. Clin. Endocrinol. Metab.* **2018**, *103*, 4043–4088. [CrossRef] [PubMed]
2. El-Maouche, D.; Arlt, W.; Merke, D.P. Congenital adrenal hyperplasia. *Lancet* **2017**, *390*, 2194–2210. [CrossRef]
3. Gidlof, S.; Falhammar, H.; Thilen, A.; von Dobeln, U.; Ritzen, M.; Wedell, A.; Nordenstrom, A. One hundred years of congenital adrenal hyperplasia in Sweden: A retrospective, population-based cohort study. *Lancet Diabetes Endocrinol.* **2013**, *1*, 35–42. [CrossRef]
4. Nordenstrom, A.; Ahmed, S.; Jones, J.; Coleman, M.; Price, D.A.; Clayton, P.E.; Hall, C.M. Female preponderance in congenital adrenal hyperplasia due to CYP21 deficiency in England: Implications for neonatal screening. *Horm. Res.* **2005**, *63*, 22–28. [CrossRef] [PubMed]
5. Falhammar, H.; Wedell, A.; Nordenstrom, A. Biochemical and genetic diagnosis of 21-hydroxylase deficiency. *Endocrine* **2015**, *50*, 306–314. [CrossRef] [PubMed]
6. Pang, S.; Hotchkiss, J.; Drash, A.L.; Levine, L.S.; New, M.I. Microfilter paper method for 17 alpha-hydroxyprogesterone radioimmunoassay: Its application for rapid screening for congenital adrenal hyperplasia. *J. Clin. Endocrinol. Metab.* **1977**, *45*, 1003–1008. [CrossRef] [PubMed]
7. White, P.C. Neonatal screening for congenital adrenal hyperplasia. *Nat. Rev. Endocrinol.* **2009**, *5*, 490–498. [CrossRef] [PubMed]
8. Van der Kamp, H.J.; Oudshoorn, C.G.; Elvers, B.H.; van Baarle, M.; Otten, B.J.; Wit, J.M.; Verkerk, P.H. Cutoff levels of 17-alpha-hydroxyprogesterone in neonatal screening for congenital adrenal hyperplasia should be based on gestational age rather than on birth weight. *J. Clin. Endocrinol. Metab.* **2005**, *90*, 3904–3907. [CrossRef] [PubMed]
9. Olgemoller, B.; Roscher, A.A.; Liebl, B.; Fingerhut, R. Screening for congenital adrenal hyperplasia: Adjustment of 17-hydroxyprogesterone cut-off values to both age and birth weight markedly improves the predictive value. *J. Clin. Endocrinol. Metab.* **2003**, *88*, 5790–5794. [CrossRef] [PubMed]
10. Allen, D.B.; Hoffman, G.L.; Fitzpatrick, P.; Laessig, R.; Maby, S.; Slyper, A. Improved precision of newborn screening for congenital adrenal hyperplasia using weight-adjusted criteria for 17-hydroxyprogesterone levels. *J. Pediatr.* **1997**, *130*, 128–133. [CrossRef]

11. Pode-Shakked, N.; Blau, A.; Pode-Shakked, B.; Tiosano, D.; Weintrob, N.; Eyal, O.; Zung, A.; Levy-Khademi, F.; Tenenbaum-Rakover, Y.; Zangen, D.; et al. Combined Gestational Age- and Birth Weight-Adjusted Cutoffs for Newborn Screening of Congenital Adrenal Hyperplasia. *J. Clin. Endocrinol. Metab.* **2019**, *104*, 3172–3180. [CrossRef] [PubMed]
12. Minutti, C.Z.; Lacey, J.M.; Magera, M.J.; Hahn, S.H.; McCann, M.; Schulze, A.; Cheillan, D.; Dorche, C.; Chace, D.H.; Lymp, J.F.; et al. Steroid profiling by tandem mass spectrometry improves the positive predictive value of newborn screening for congenital adrenal hyperplasia. *J. Clin. Endocrinol. Metab.* **2004**, *89*, 3687–3693. [CrossRef] [PubMed]
13. Janzen, N.; Peter, M.; Sander, S.; Steuerwald, U.; Terhardt, M.; Holtkamp, U.; Sander, J. Newborn screening for congenital adrenal hyperplasia: Additional steroid profile using liquid chromatography-tandem mass spectrometry. *J. Clin. Endocrinol. Metab.* **2007**, *92*, 2581–2589. [CrossRef] [PubMed]
14. Krone, N.; Arlt, W. Genetics of congenital adrenal hyperplasia. *Best Pr. Res. Clin. Endocrinol. Metab.* **2009**, *23*, 181–192. [CrossRef] [PubMed]
15. Wedell, A. Molecular genetics of 21-hydroxylase deficiency. *Endocr. Dev.* **2011**, *20*, 80–87. [PubMed]
16. Thil'en, A.; Nordenstrom, A.; Hagenfeldt, L.; von Dobeln, U.; Guthenberg, C.; Larsson, A. Benefits of neonatal screening for congenital adrenal hyperplasia (21-hydroxylase deficiency) in Sweden. *Pediatrics* **1998**, *101*, E11. [CrossRef] [PubMed]
17. Gidlof, S.; Wedell, A.; Guthenberg, C.; von Dobeln, U.; Nordenstrom, A. Nationwide neonatal screening for congenital adrenal hyperplasia in sweden: A 26-year longitudinal prospective population-based study. *JAMA Pediatr.* **2014**, *168*, 567–574. [CrossRef] [PubMed]
18. Nordenstrom, A.; Falhammar, H. Management of Endocrine Disease: Diagnosis and management of the patient with non-classic CAH due to 21-hydroxylase deficiency. *Eur. J. Endocrinol.* **2019**, *180*, R127–R145. [CrossRef] [PubMed]
19. Kohn, B.; Day, D.; Alemzadeh, R.; Enerio, D.; Patel, S.V.; Pelczar, J.V.; Speiser, P.W. Splicing mutation in CYP21 associated with delayed presentation of salt-wasting congenital adrenal hyperplasia. *Am. J. Med. Genet.* **1995**, *57*, 450–454. [CrossRef] [PubMed]
20. Boelen, A.; Ruiter, A.F.; Claahsen-van der Grinten, H.L.; Endert, E.; Ackermans, M.T. Determination of a steroid profile in heel prick blood using LC-MS/MS. *Bioanalysis* **2016**, *8*, 375–384. [CrossRef] [PubMed]

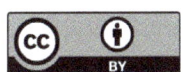

© 2020 by the authors. Licensee MDPI, Basel, Switzerland. This article is an open access article distributed under the terms and conditions of the Creative Commons Attribution (CC BY) license (http://creativecommons.org/licenses/by/4.0/).

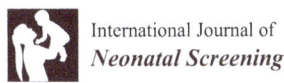

Article

Landscape of Congenital Adrenal Hyperplasia Newborn Screening in the United States

Sari Edelman *, Hiral Desai, Trey Pigg, Careema Yusuf and Jelili Ojodu

Association of Public Health Laboratories, Silver Spring, MD 20910, USA; hiral.desai@aphl.org (H.D.); trey.pigg@aphl.org (T.P.); careema.yusuf@aphl.org (C.Y.); jelili.ojodu@aphl.org (J.O.)
* Correspondence: sari.edelman@aphl.org

Received: 8 June 2020; Accepted: 11 August 2020; Published: 14 August 2020

Abstract: Newborn screening (NBS) is a state-based public health program that aims to identify newborns at risk of certain disorders in the first days after birth to prevent permanent disability or death. Disorders on the Health and Human Services Federal Advisory Committee's Recommended Uniform Screening Panel (RUSP) have been adopted by most state NBS programs; however, each state mandates specific disorders to be screened and implements their own system processes. Congenital adrenal hyperplasia (CAH) was added to the RUSP in 2005, and currently all 53 NBS programs universally screen for it. This paper provides a landscape of CAH screening in the United States, utilizing data voluntarily entered by state NBS programs in the Newborn Screening Technical assistance and Evaluation Program data repository. Data reported encompasses NBS state profile data (follow-up, disorder testing and the reporting of processes and methodologies for screening), quality indicator data (timeliness of CAH NBS) and confirmed cases. This comprehensive landscape analysis compares the CAH NBS systems across the US. This is vital in ultimately ensuring that newborns with CAH at risk of salt crisis receive appropriate intervention in a timely manner.

Keywords: newborn screening; congenital adrenal hyperplasia; NewSTEPs

1. Introduction

Newborn screening (NBS) is a state-based public health program that aims to identify newborns at risk for certain disorders in the first days or weeks after birth, in order to prevent permanent disability or death. The US Health and Human Services (HHS) Federal Advisory Committee on Heritable Disorders in Newborns and Children (ACHDNC) evaluates and recommends disorders to be included in the Recommended Uniform Screening Panel (RUSP). However, each state mandates the specific disorders to be screened by their own program, implements system processes including the follow-up of out-of-range (screen-positive) results, and is responsible for the quality improvement and assurance of the entire NBS system [1].

This paper provides a landscape of congenital adrenal hyperplasia (CAH) screening in the United States, utilizing data voluntarily entered by state NBS programs in the Newborn Screening Technical Assistance and Evaluation Program (NewSTEPs) data repository.

By the time CAH was added to the RUSP in 2005, 72% ($n = 38/53$) of NBS programs were already universally screening for the disorder. Of NBS programs, 19% ($n = 10/53$) implemented universal screening for CAH in 2005 or after, and 9% ($n = 5/53$) of NBS programs did not know or did not have access to that year of implementation information. Currently, all 53 NBS programs universally screen for CAH, programs which consist of the 50 US states, the District of Columbia, Puerto Rico and Guam (Figure 1). CAH, caused by steroid 21-hydroxylase deficiency, occurs in 1/15,000 births, and is more common in certain populations [2]. NewSTEPs collects and classifies CAH cases in three categories: Classic 21-hydroxylase deficiency (salt-wasting), Classic 21-hydroxylase deficiency (simple virilizing), and other adrenal disorder. By identifying babies with severe, salt-wasting CAH before they develop adrenal crises, screening reduces morbidity and mortality, especially among affected boys. Diagnosis is based on elevated levels of 17-hydroxyprogesterone (17-OHP), the preferred substrate for steroid 21-hydroxylase [3].

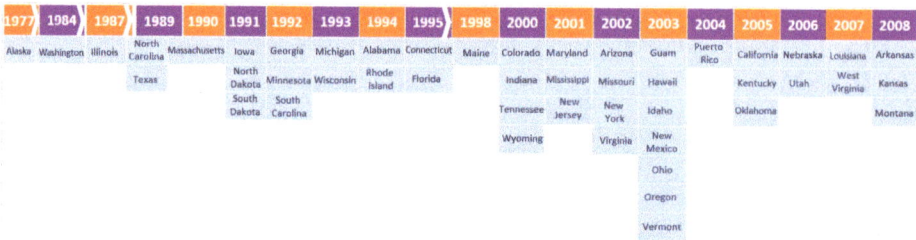

Figure 1. Timeline of congenital adrenal hyperplasia (CAH) newborn screening implementation in the United States.

2. Materials and Methods

2.1. NewSTEPs State Profiles

NewSTEPs [4], a program of the Association of Public Health Laboratories (APHL), is the national NBS resource center designed to provide data, technical assistance and training to US NBS programs and assist them with quality improvement initiatives. It functions with the goal of improving outcomes for newborns by facilitating NBS initiatives and programmatic outcomes, including the offering of expertise in NBS program development and evaluation, member connection and data analysis to improve the overall quality of the NBS system [5]. Aligning with this goal, NewSTEPs maintains a centralized and secure data repository that is designed to collect comprehensive data on NBS programs. The data collected encompass NBS state profile data (public facing, programmatic overview data), quality indicator data (restricted to authorized users, metrics of program performance) and confirmed cases (restricted to authorized users). NewSTEPs collects individual-level confirmed case data, as well as aggregate counts of confirmed cases by NBS programs. While registration for the repository is open to all who are interested, restricted data elements, which include confirmed cases and quality indicators, are only accessible to individuals who are granted data access and data entry permissions by each NBS program. NewSTEPs requires that NBS programs have a signed Memorandum of Understanding (MOU) with APHL in order to enter restricted data elements. This manuscript includes state profile data from all 53 NBS programs in the US, as well as individual-level case data from 35 NBS programs with signed MOUs. This manuscript refers to non-CAH cases as all cases from the RUSP, excluding CAH, which have been entered into the NewSTEPs data repository.

NewSTEPs collects data in accordance with an established data entry timeline [6]. NBS programs are encouraged to update state profile and quality indicator data on an annual basis, and case data from two years prior on an annual basis. This is to accommodate for the time it takes to resolve and close out cases. Individual-level CAH cases adhere to a set of public health surveillance case definitions that have been developed by the NBS community to facilitate common classifications for diagnoses across programs (see Supplementary Materials for NewSTEPs' CAH case definition). Consensus public health surveillance case definitions for NBS disorders allow for the consistent categorization and tracking of newborns identified with disorders [7].

2.2. CAH Data Request

NewSTEPs followed the formal policies and procedures established for requesting case-level data for use in this paper. The request for data was channeled through APHL's governance structure and directed to the Data Review Workgroup, which is charged with providing expertise in order to make recommendations to NewSTEPs staff and the NewSTEPs Steering Committee on any requests made for data collected within the repository. The Data Review Workgroup has no objections to the use of data presented in this paper.

State profile data are represented as of March 2020. In total, 53 NBS programs contribute state profile data, however not all programs contribute data to all fields. NBS programs reporting individual case data ($N = 35$) are represented from 2015 to 2017 to align with the NewSTEPs' data entry timeline.

2.3. CAH Data Query and Analytics

In addition to routine data submission efforts (customized technical assistance, interactive Tableau data visualizations, phone and email reminders of data entry timeline, customized tutorials of the NewSTEPs website and data repository, user guides and reports of frequently asked questions, and import templates and other tools to facilitate data entry), NBS program-specific encrypted CSV files were sent to NBS program case data entry staff with instruction to review fields to ease the data submission of requested missing fields of cases entered. The analyzed CAH case data fields in this report included gestational age, birth weight, biological sex, societal sex, family history, final diagnosis, mutational analysis, 17-OHP serum levels and timeliness intervals for CAH screening. The number of missing fields were specific to each program. These fields were selected as they offered the most quantitative and qualitative data to allow for a sufficient landscape of CAH screening.

These efforts were followed up with targeted phone outreach. Efforts were successful in cleaning data and updating missing fields, however not all missing fields were updated due to programs not collecting or not having certain information. Data were queried from the repository using a combination of Structure Query Language (SQL) and Tableau. Open source libraries and statistical functions from R 3.6.3 were utilized to analyze data and explore dataset patterns by parsing elements queried from the NewSTEPs data repository.

3. Results

3.1. State Profile Data

One screen vs. two screen: Each state or territory has mandates to screen newborns, and these mandates specify if newborns will receive one or two screens. Thirteen states (Alabama, Arizona, Colorado, Delaware, Idaho, Maryland, Nevada, New Mexico, Oregon, Texas, Utah, Washington and Wyoming) are considered two-screen states, because they require that a second dried blood spot (DBS) specimen be collected on all newborns regardless of the results of the first newborn screen. Newborns in the other 40 states and territories typically undergo a single newborn screen. If a specimen is collected too early, or if there is an unsatisfactory specimen due to collection or transport errors, an additional screen may be prompted [1].

Short-term follow-up: Of the NBS Programs, 62% ($n = 33$) define short-term follow-up in their state as until a diagnosis is made or ruled out; 21% ($n = 11$) define it as until the baby is on treatment; 4% ($n = 2$) define it as until confirmatory testing is performed; 13% ($n = 7$) define it as other. Other responses included a combination of until diagnosis is made or ruled out, or the baby is on treatment ($n = 3$); a combination of until confirmatory testing is performed, or the baby has seen a specialist, is on treatment or the diagnosis is made or ruled out ($n = 3$); and a breakdown of short-term follow-up of borderline (until diagnosis is made and ruled out, or three months) versus presumptive positive (until diagnosis is made and ruled out, or one year) ($n = 1$). Although the Clinical and Laboratory Standards Institute (CLSI) does not define short-term follow-up specifically, follow-up is defined as actions taken to ensure that a person whose test results are screen positive or invalid receives appropriate further tests and evaluation in a timely fashion, and as actions taken that ensure the newborn screening system evaluates the effectiveness of screening [8].

Time-critical disorder screening and reporting out processes: CAH is considered a time-critical disorder [9]. One hundred percent of NBS programs that provided data ($n = 49/49$) run tests for time-critical disorders, inclusive of CAH testing, five days of the week on Monday through Friday. Sixty-seven percent ($n = 33/49$) run tests for time-critical disorders on Saturday, 20% ($n = 10/49$) on Sunday, and 51% ($n = 25/49$) during holidays (Figure 2). All of the NBS programs ($n = 49/49$) report on time-critical disorders Monday to Friday. Sixty-three percent ($n = 31/49$) carry out tests on Saturday; 33% ($n = 16/49$) carry out tests on Sunday; and, 57% ($n = 28/49$) carry out tests on holidays (Figure 2).

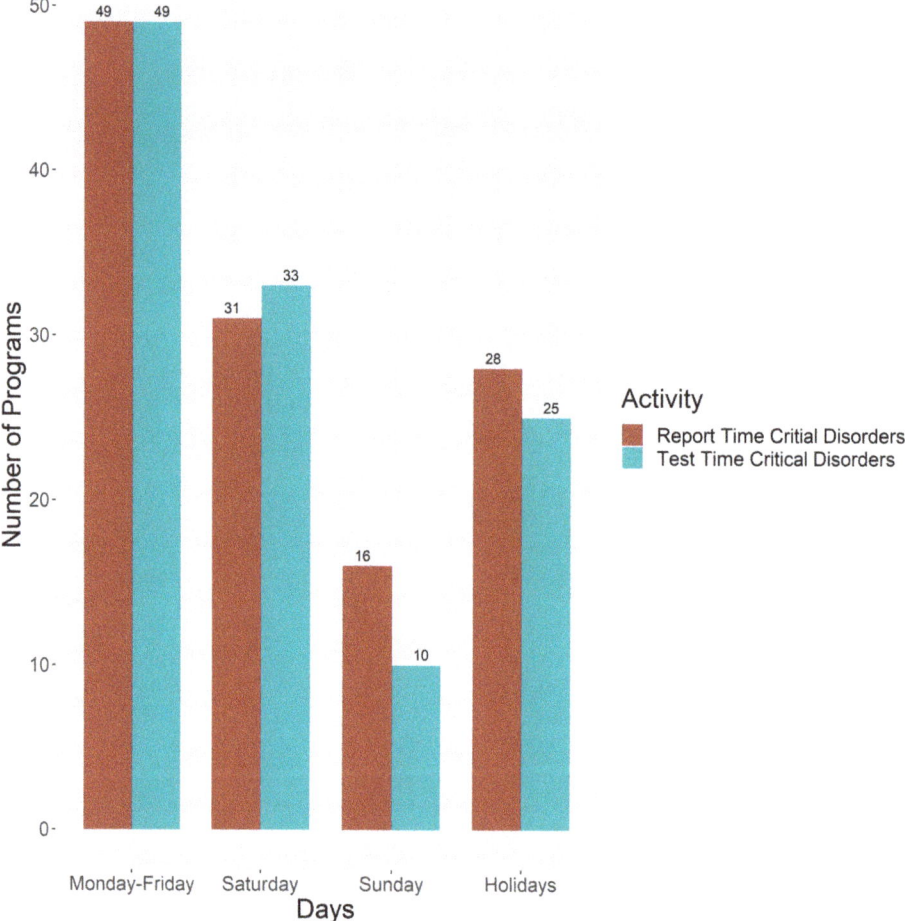

Figure 2. Days newborn screening (NBS) laboratories test for time-critical disorders and days NBS offer follow-up reports on time-critical disorders ($N = 49$).

3.2. Methodology for Screening

All 53 NBS programs screen for CAH using fully integrated fluoroimmunoassay (FIA) as their first screen method, with 17-OHP as the target. Twenty-nine programs use the PerkinElmer Genetic Screening Processor (GSP) for first tier screening, while the remaining 24 programs use the PerkinElmer AutoDELFIA instrument. Both instruments apply the same immunoreaction technology and have the same reagents to measure 17-OHP, however the GSP is a newer model with higher throughput.

Eleven NBS programs provided first-screen, second tier methodology and target data for CAH. Six NBS programs reported also using FIA for their second tier, and five NBS programs extracted 17-OHP specifically. Four NBS programs reported using liquid chromatography tandem mass spectrometry (LC-MS/MS) for their second tier, with a combination of 17-OHP ($n = 4$), adrostenedione ($n = 2$), cortisol ($n = 2$), 17-OHP + adrostenedione/cortisol ($n = 2$), 11-Deoxycorticosterone ($n = 1$) and 21-Deoxycortisol ($n = 2$) as the screening target (programs can enter multiple screening targets). The remaining program reported sending specimens for second tier screening to Mayo Clinic Laboratories.

3.3. Confirmed Case Data

NewSTEPs collects individual-level confirmed cases in the NewSTEPs data repository in accordance with public health surveillance case definitions, as well as aggregate case counts per condition. From the years 2015 to 2017, 495 individual-level cases were entered by 35 participating NBS programs. Comparatively, 10,892 individual non-CAH cases were entered by 36 participating NBS programs. Furthermore, 826 aggregate case counts of CAH were entered from 49 participating NBS programs within the same timeframe.

Gestational age and birth weight: The median gestational age of individual-level CAH cases entered ($N = 222$) was 39 weeks, with an interquartile range (IQR) of 37–40 weeks. This was the same as the median gestational age of all non-CAH cases entered in the data repository ($N = 6531$). The median birth weight of CAH cases entered ($N = 222$) was 3317.5 g with an IQR of 2976.5–3700 g. Similarly, the median birth weight of all non-CAH cases entered in the data repository was 3180 grams ($N = 10,015$). Figures 3 and 4 show the distribution of gestational age and birth weight. The median birth weight for 262 male infants was 3371.5, with an IQR of 2975.5–3757.25 grams; the median birth weight for 203 females was 3270 with an IQR of 2955–3577.5 grams. The p-value of 0.03 indicates that the differences in the distribution of male and female birth weight are statistically significant.

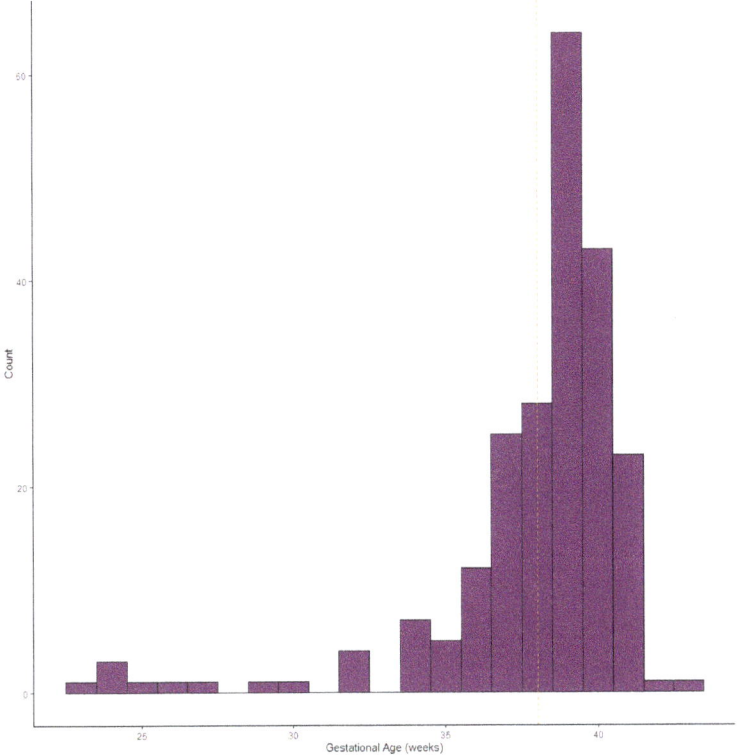

Figure 3. Congenital adrenal hyperplasia cases: distribution of gestational age ($N = 222$).

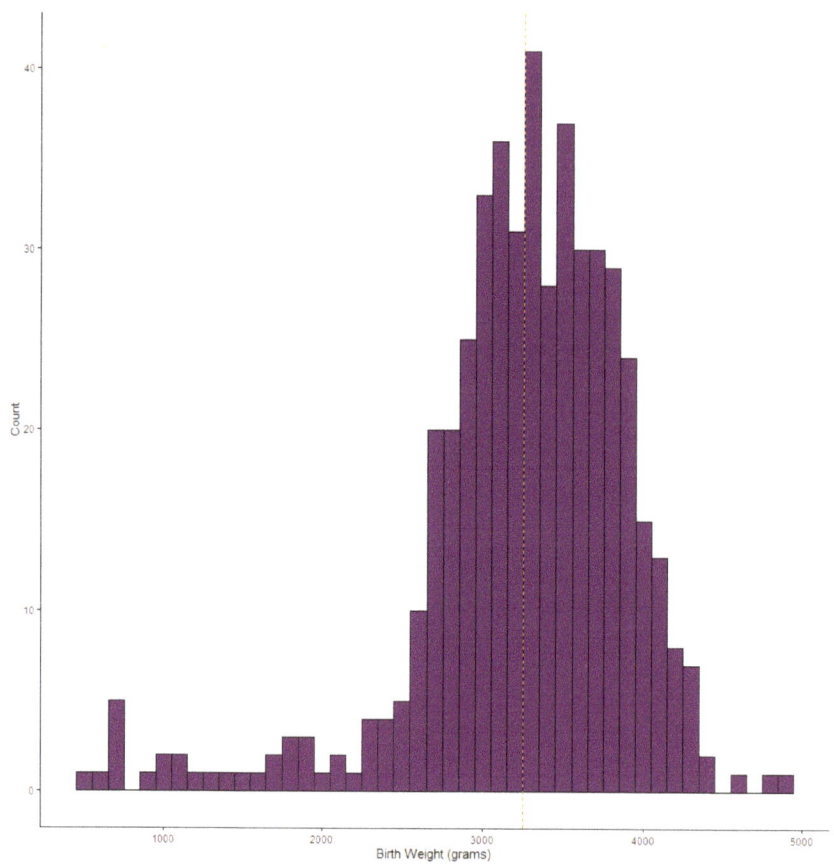

Figure 4. Congenital adrenal hyperplasia cases: distribution of birth weight ($N = 484$).

3.4. Diagnostic Workup Data

Final diagnosis: Of these cases, 37% ($n = 185/495$) had a final diagnosis of Classic 21-hydroxylase deficiency (salt-wasting); 6% ($n = 31/495$) had a final diagnosis of Classic 21-hydroxylase deficiency (simple virilizing); 6% ($n = 27/495$) had a final diagnosis of other adrenal disorder, and 51% ($n = 252/495$) did not provide sufficient data to classify the type of CAH. The distribution of phenotypes by final diagnosis did not vary considerably year to year.

17-OHP Serum Levels: The 17-OHP serum level ranges can be observed in Figure 5 from a total of 232 entered cases, and include levels reported as "unknown" or "untested." Data was not reported for 263 cases. Of the 232 cases entered, 33.2% ($n = 77$) of 17-OHP serum levels were between 1000 and 10,000 ng/dL, 29.7% ($n = 69$) were greater than 10,000 ng/dL, and 9.9% ($n = 23$) were less than 1000 ng/dL (Figure 5).

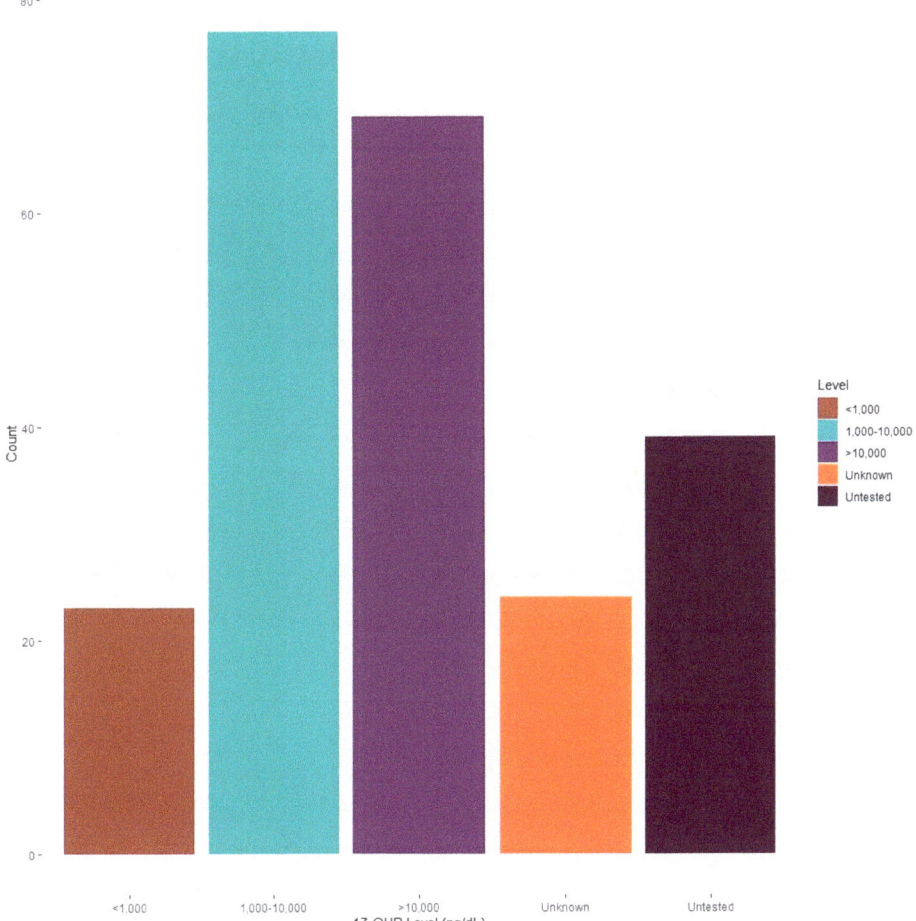

Figure 5. Congenital adrenal hyperplasia cases: 17-OHP serum levels ($N = 232$).

According to the American College of Obstetricians and Gynecologists and the Society for Maternal Fetal Medicine, a pregnancy is considered early term at 37 weeks of gestation through 38 6/7 weeks of gestation, and full term at 39 weeks of gestation through 40 6/7 weeks of gestation [10]. Of the 77 cases that had 17-OHP levels between 1000 and 10,000 ng/dL, the gestational age was between 25 and 38 weeks for 24 infants, 39 and 40 weeks for 35 infants, it was 41 weeks for 8 infants and was unreported for 10 infants. One case indicated a 17-OHP level less than 1000 ng/dL, but reported an actual value of 627 ng/dL with a final diagnosis of Classic 21-hydroxylase deficiency (salt-wasting). The gestational age for this infant was 39 weeks. Of the 23 cases that reported 17-OHP levels less than 1000 ng/dL, 6 infants' gestational ages were between 32 and 38 weeks, 7 infants' gestational ages were between 39 and 40 weeks, 3 infants' gestational ages were between 41 and 43 weeks, and data was not reported for 7 infants.

Biological and societal sex: According to NewSTEPs, biological sex is determined at the birthing facility and included on the dried blood spot card, while societal sex is determined during the diagnostic process. Of the 203 cases entered with a female biological sex, 33% ($n = 67$) also had a female societal sex and 67% ($n = 136$) had an unknown or unspecified societal sex, or did not provide data on societal sex. Of the 263 cases entered with a male biological sex, 38% ($n = 101$) also had a male societal sex, 0.4% ($n = 1$) had a female societal sex and 61% ($n = 161$) had an unknown or unspecified societal sex, or did not provide data on societal sex. Of the 11 cases entered with no data on biological sex, 9% ($n = 1$) had a male societal sex, and 91% ($n = 10$) did not provide data on societal sex. Of the 18 cases entered with unknown or unspecified biological sex, 33% ($n = 6$) had a female societal sex, 6% ($n = 1$) had a male societal sex and 61% ($n = 11$) had an unknown or unspecified societal sex, or did not provide data on societal sex.

Out of the cases that did report biological sex, Classic 21-hydroxylase deficiency (salt-wasting) was the most common final diagnosis amongst females ($n = 66$), males ($n = 104$) and infants with unknown or unspecified biological sex ($n = 14$), whereas another adrenal disorder was the most common final diagnosis amongst those cases for whom data was provided on biological sex ($n = 4$; Figure 6).

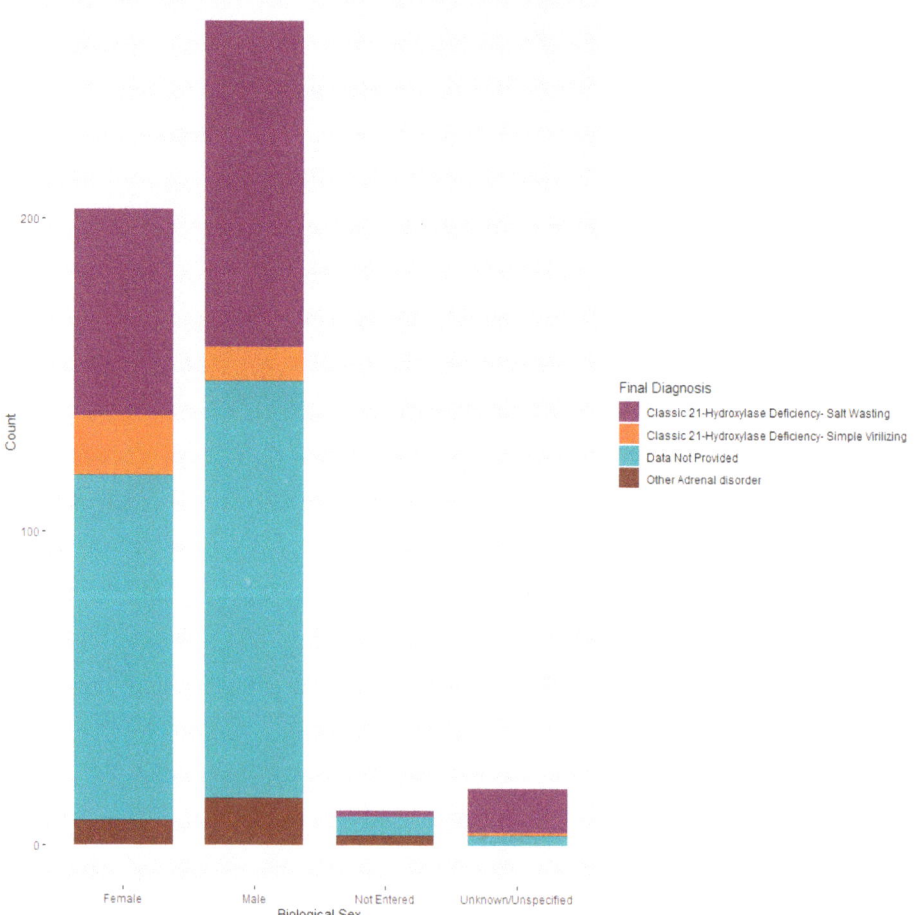

Figure 6. Congenital adrenal hyperplasia cases: final diagnosis by biological sex from 2015 to 2017 ($N = 495$).

3.5. Timeliness Data

Initial specimen collection: The recommendations for initial specimen collection are between 24 and 48 h after birth in every state NBS program, except for California [11]. The median time for specimen collection ($N = 482$) between 2015 and 2017 was 31 h, with an IQR of 24.5–39 h (Figure 7). A one-sample t-test was used, and showed a p-value of 6.7×10^{-7}, which is less than the significance level of 0.05. The plot below visualizes density, indicating that most specimens were collected between 24 and 30 h of birth. Specimen collection time did not vary considerably from 2015 to 2017.

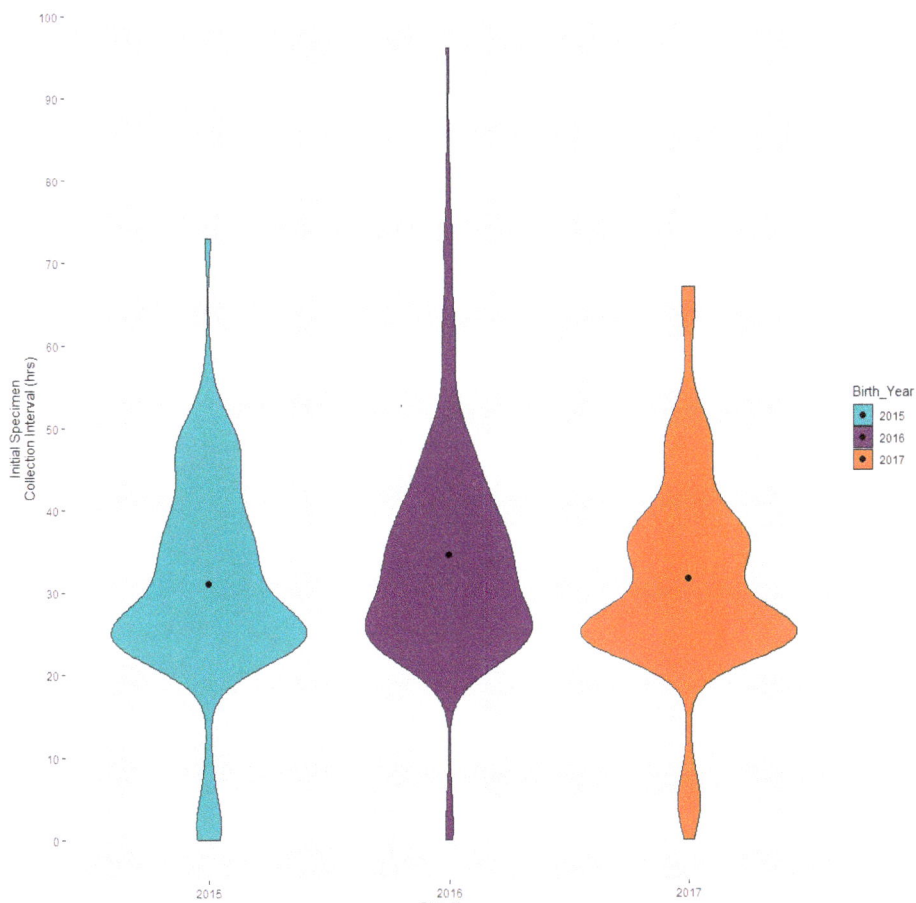

Figure 7. Congenital adrenal hyperplasia cases: time from birth to specimen collection in hours ($N = 478$).

Specimen receipt interval: The median time from birth to receipt of the specimens by the laboratory was 3 days, with an IQR of 3–4 days ($N = 470$). The specimen receipt interval remained similar from 2015 to 2017. The p-value of 0.17 indicates that there is no significant change in specimen receipt interval through the years.

Initial specimen result release: The median time from birth to release of out-of-range CAH results ($N = 453$) was 4 days, with an IQR of 3–6 days (Figure 8). Comparatively, the median release of out-of-range non-CAH results (N = 9564) from birth was 6 days. The *p*-value of 0.12 indicates that there was no significant reduciton in initial result release.

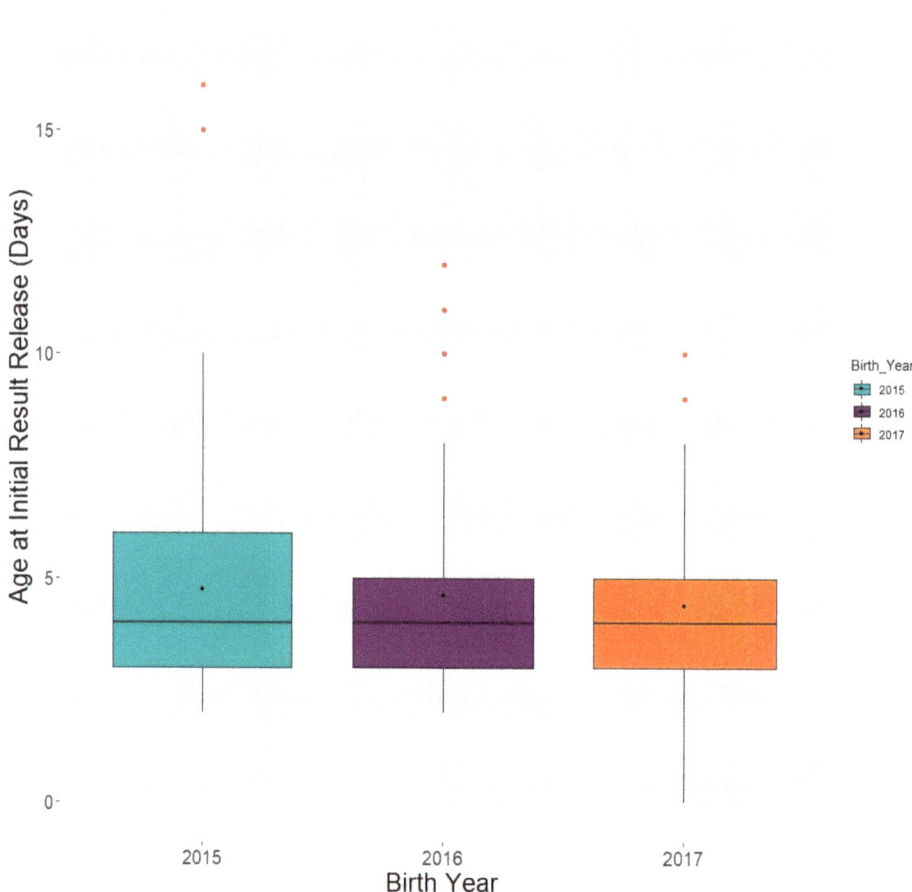

Figure 8. Congenital adrenal hyperplasia cases: time interval from birth to release of out-of-range results (N = 453).

3.6. Subsequent Specimen Collection

Subsequent specimen collection: NewSTEPs defines a subsequent specimen as any specimen received at the laboratory for a given newborn screen after the first specimen has been received. A subsequent specimen may be requested based on a borderline result from the first specimen, or an unacceptable first specimen. There may be multiple subsequent specimens per screen [12]. The median for subsequent specimen collection (N = 287) was 13 days of life, with an IQR of 8–16 days. (Figure 9). The *p*-value of 0.74 indicated that subsequent specimen collection through the years has not significantly changed.

Subsequent specimen receipt interval: The median time from birth to subsequent specimen receipt at laboratory (N = 287) was 16.1 days, with an IQR of 10–20 days. The *p*-value of 0.44 indicated that there was no real change in subsequent specimen receipt interval from 2015 to 2017.

Subsequent specimen receipt result release interval: The median age of the infant at subsequent specimen receipt of out-of-range CAH results was 19 days ($N = 287$; Figure 10). The p-value 0.85 showed that there was not a significant change in the result release interval from 2015 to 2017. In comparison, the median time interval of the subsequent specimen release of out-of-range non-CAH results ($N = 3877$) from birth was 17 days.

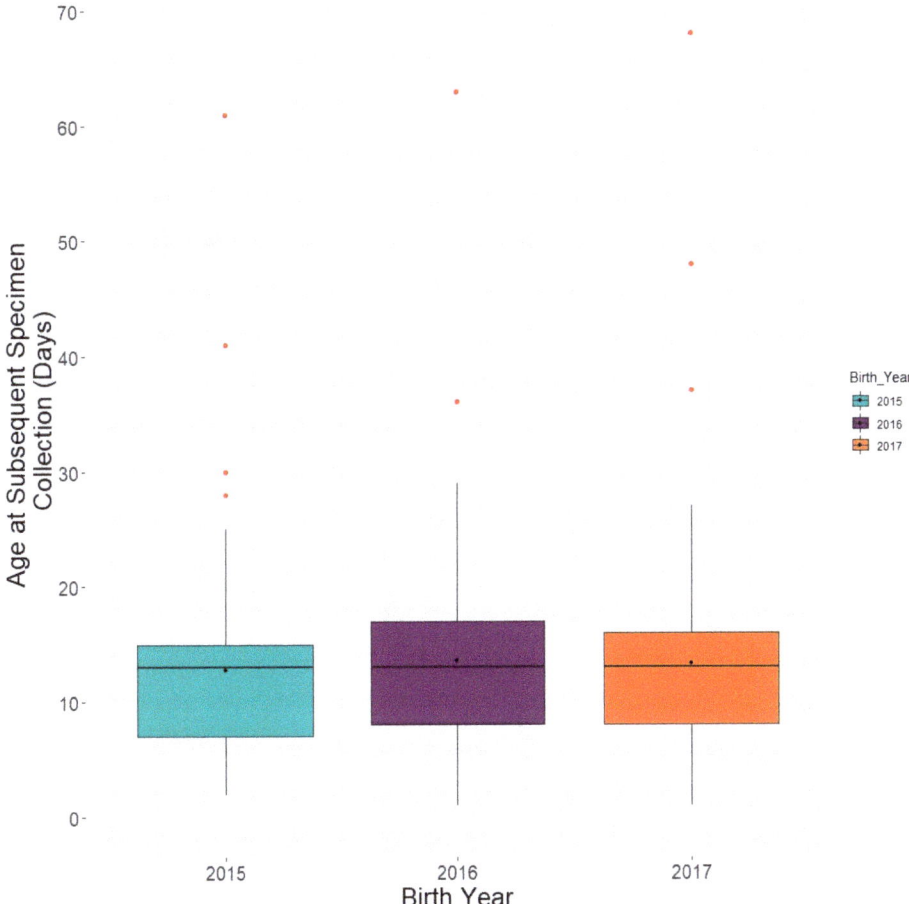

Figure 9. Congenital adrenal hyperplasia cases: age at subsequent specimen collection ($N = 287$).

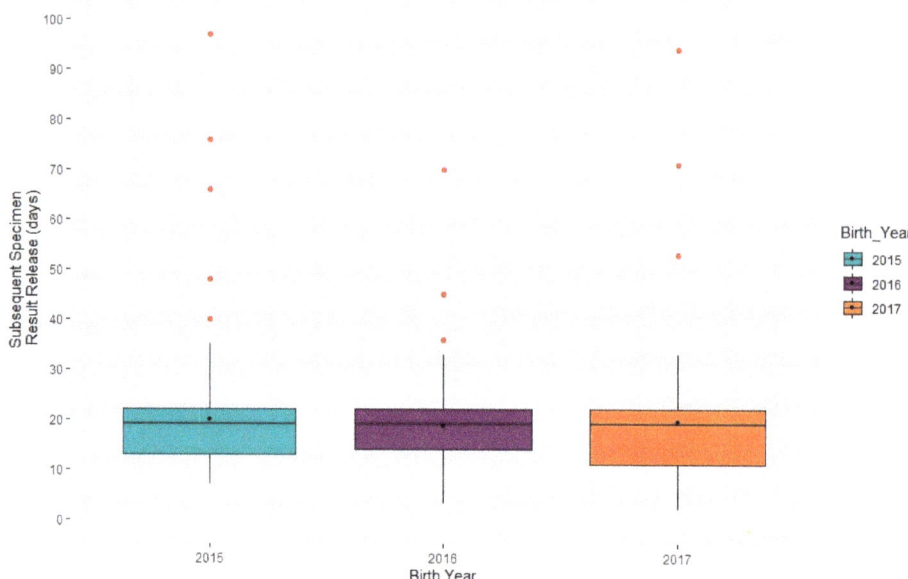

Figure 10. Congenital adrenal hyperplasia cases: subsequent specimen result release of out-of-range results, by year (*N* = 287).

NewSTEPs defines intervention by an appropriate medical provider as the date of the clinic visit or hospital consultation to evaluate the potential diagnosis of CAH [13]. The median time from birth to intervention by an appropriate medical provider for CAH cases (*N* = 233) was 6 days. The median time from birth to intervention for all non-CAH cases (*N* = 6713) was 13 days. The median time from birth to confirmation of diagnosis of CAH cases (*N* = 243) was 10 days (Figure 11). The p-values of 0.12 and 0.31 indicated that there were no significant changes in the time to intervention or diagnosis, respectively, for CAH cases screened from 2015 to 2017. The median time from birth to confirmation of diagnosis was also 10 days for the CAH cases submitted by the 13 NBS programs who entered data for all three years. Comparatively, the median time from birth to confirmation of diagnosis for all non-CAH cases (*N* = 7505) was 24 days.

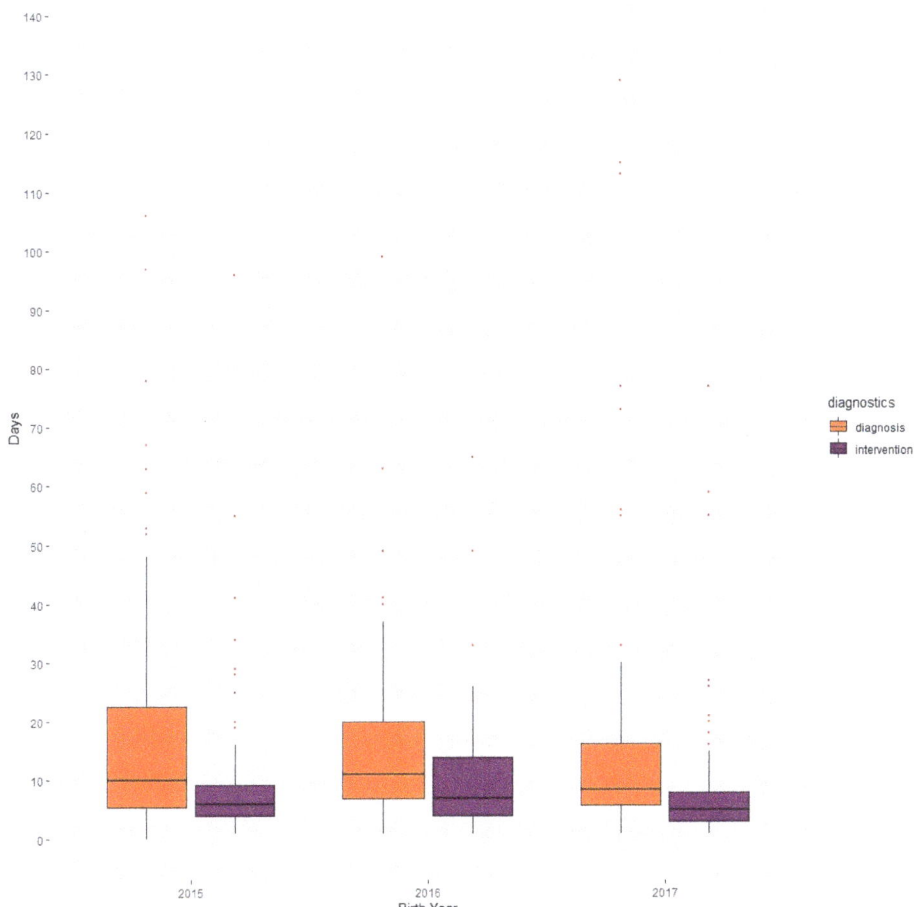

Figure 11. Congenital adrenal hyperplasia cases: time interval from birth to intervention and confirmation of diagnosis, by year.

4. Discussion

4.1. State Profile Data

While most NBS programs are considered one-screen states, there are certain circumstances, such as if a specimen is collected too early or if there is an unsatisfactory specimen due to collection or transport errors, that may prompt an additional screen. A 2015 study indicated that there is no clear consensus among state NBS programs on whether the routine second screening of newborns can identify clinically relevant cases of CAH [14].

Although NBS programs define short-term follow-up differently, every program conducts follow-ups on infants at risk of having an NBS disorder. Most programs define short-term follow-up in their state as until a diagnosis is made or ruled out. Furthermore, NBS programs differ in hours of operation depending on day of the week. Certain activities may be prioritized or not conducted at all, depending on state-specific standard operating procedures. However, all NBS programs run tests for and report on results for time-critical disorders Monday to Friday. It should be noted that 16 NBS programs have laboratories that are open five days a week, 26 are open six days a week, and 11 are open seven days a week. A recent publication found that laboratory operating hours are a critical factor associated with timeliness, and that infants receiving services independent of the day of the week they were born will show a reduced risk of tragic outcomes for their individual families [15].

All NBS programs screen for CAH using FIA as their first screen method, with 17-OHP as the target. About half of the programs use the PerkinElmer GSP, and the other half use the PerkinElmer AutoDELFIA instrument. For the second tier, about half of the programs reporting data use FIA, and the other use LC-MS/MS with varying method targets.

4.2. Confirmed Case Data

NBS programs report the number of aggregate cases of each disorder on the RUSP identified by DBS NBS to the NewSTEPs data repository. For the years 2015, 2016 and 2017, there has been a total of 826 aggregate case counts of CAH from 49 participating NBS programs, as of March 2020.

NBS programs also report confirmed infant-level case data to the NewSTEPs data repository. From the years 2015–2017, 495 individual cases were entered in the data repository from 35 participating NBS programs. It should be noted that state participation per year varied. For example, the number of state NBS programs contributing data are different in 2015 than in 2016 and 2017. There are several reasons for this discrepancy between aggregate and individual cases in the NewSTEPs data repository. First, not all NBS programs are able to provide all required fields for individual case entry, specifically diagnostic workup data. NBS programs may not have received this information back from physicians or specialists, or may have restrictions on the level of data they can report to NewSTEPs and outside organizations. Furthermore, NBS programs may not collect the level of data that NewSTEPs requests, such as some of the demographic fields (gestational age, and biological and societal sex). Barriers to data entry include data entry staff shortages, high turnovers of staff and a lack of NewSTEPs integration into workflows. Although NewSTEPs adheres to a data entry timeline, performs numerous methods of targeted outreach to state NBS programs for data collection and strives to ease and automate this process, all data entered in the repository is voluntary.

Almost all NBS programs were able to provide data on birth weight, however gestational age data proved more difficult, with 45% ($n = 222/495$) of all cases entered providing this data. Reasons reported for this include the following: no demographic data was available, previous laboratory information management systems did not capture this data, some cases were reported to the NBS program with missing data, and NBS programs are unable to report gestational age or do not collect gestational age. There was no difference in median gestational age or median birth weight among CAH cases and non-CAH cases, indicating that having CAH does not impact these factors.

Affected females with CAH may have ambiguous genitalia that alert medical professionals at the clinical level to their condition, and prompt appropriate diagnosis and treatment. In particular, affected females with Classic 21-hydroxylase deficiency (simple virilizing) are most often diagnosed immediately at birth, whereas affected males present with normal male genitalia, and thus their condition is detected at the prenatal or newborn screening level [16]. There was one instance in the repository in which societal sex differed from biological sex entered. There were eight additional instances in which no data was provided on biological sex, or it was unknown or unspecified, and societal sex was reported. It is possible that additional cases exist with incorrect initial sex assignation at birth. However, NewSTEPs does not collect long-term follow-up data, which is needed for this analysis. Of the information provided, in males, females and infants with unknown or unspecified biological sex, the final diagnosis was most commonly reported as Classic 21-hydroxylase deficiency (salt-wasting). This is in line with recent journal findings [17]. However, of the cases that did not provide data on biological sex, only one case had this as the final diagnosis; the remainder were identified as other adrenal disorders or data was not provided. Long-term follow-up data and complete diagnostic data are necessary for the further analysis of biological and societal sex among CAH cases.

Despite the high null value for 17-OHP serum level reporting, most programs reported levels between 1000 and 10,000 ng/dL, followed by levels greater than 10,000 ng/dL. While types of CAH cases are categorized by NBS programs, NewSTEPs public health surveillance case definitions classify them into either definite, probable or possible. According to these definitions, 17-OHP serum levels between 1000 and 10,000 ng/dL have a greater likelihood of being probable cases of CAH, while serum levels greater than 10,000 have a greater likelihood of being definite cases [18]. There is a need for more complete clinical diagnostic information, particularly for those cases that do not fit within the typical reference range for CAH, in order to determine whether other interferences may have altered NBS values. Despite the high null value for phenotypes supplied by final diagnosis due to the aforementioned barriers, most individual cases entered into the NewSTEPs data repository had a final diagnosis of Classic 21-hydroxylase deficiency (salt-wasting). Final diagnoses of other adrenal disorders and Classic 21-hydroxylase deficiency (simple virilizing) had approximately the same numbers of cases entered. Studies have shown that gestational age is a better predictor of 17-OHP levels in newborns with CAH, and may guide the interpretation of screening results [19].

A recently published journal article noted the final status of CAH cases not being reported to state laboratories, and the need for quality improvement efforts to be directed at enhanced communication between clinicians and state laboratories, in addition to transparent reporting of states' efforts on a national platform [17]. NewSTEPs data is in accordance with this finding, as NBS programs receive diagnoses back, but not necessarily detailed diagnostic level information. Other incomplete diagnostic workup fields, including mutation analysis data, further emphasize the need for more robust data collection. NewSTEPs does help with this effort and with quality improvement processes within state NBS programs.

4.3. Timeliness Data

The median time of hours from birth to specimen collection for cases between 2015 and 2017 stayed within the 24–48 h collection timeframe recommended by the ACHDNC [11]. The median time of specimen collection did not vary considerably year to year, indicating that the NBS programs are performing well within this metric, although there is room for quality improvement. Thirty-three specimens were collected prior to 24 h of collection, which are deemed unsatisfactory specimens by NBS programs. Individual programs decide whether or not to screen these or wait for a subsequent specimen.

Similarly, the median time of 4 days for CAH results being reported falls within the ACDHNC's timeliness recommendation of time-critical results being reported within five days of life. This is slightly faster than the median time of 6 days for non-CAH results being reported, which also falls within ACHDNC's timeliness recommendation of all results being reported within seven days of life. Furthermore, there were fewer results being reported after more than 5 days of life in 2017 and 2016 than in 2015. This highlights the significant efforts of NBS programs to operate their testing facilities and release out of range results as rapidly as possible. Quality improvement efforts implemented throughout NBS processes in order to sustain and improve upon timeliness metrics include the following: providing education to submitters and courier services about the importance of timely collection and shipment of specimens, expanding operating hours, improving laboratory workflows, and improving health information technology infrastructure in order to better transmit laboratory orders and results [15].

The median time for subsequent CAH results being reported was two days longer than the non-CAH results. This was an unexpected result, and further analysis is needed to determine cause.

There was no significant change in the median time interval from birth to receipt of specimens by the laboratory from 2015 to 2017. The reasons for outliers and delays in specimen receipt at the laboratory, as noted by NBS programs, included severe weather, lack of courier operations on holidays, delays in specimen shipment by midwives and the difficulty experienced by courier services in accessing rural or remote birthing facilities. Some of these challenges are being addressed by the aforementioned quality improvement efforts among NBS programs. NewSTEPs defines intervention by an appropriate medical provider as the earliest point at which a clinical action was rendered, based on the follow-up of the NBS results; this is inclusive of the date therapy was initiated or a decision was made to defer therapy based on current presentation. For CAH, it is the date of clinic visit or hospital consultation to evaluate the potential diagnosis of CAH:

- Standard confirmatory testing: Clinician draws electrolytes and 17-OHP;
- Electrolytes may or may not indicate need for urgent intervention, however a decision is rendered based on laboratory results and the clinical presentation of the infant;
- Advanced confirmatory testing: In cases in which exam or presentation strongly suggests diagnosis of CAH, additional adrenal testing may be warranted in consultation with endocrinologist.

The date of diagnosis is defined as when the diagnosis was confirmed upon elevated 17-OHP (+/− other abnormal adrenal hormone abnormalities) and evaluation by endocrinologist [13]. Fewer programs were able to report on intervention by medical provider and confirmation of diagnosis intervals. NBS programs often do not have this information, and may not receive this level of data back from clinicians. However, the median time to diagnosis and median time to intervention from data reported were not statistically significant, suggesting that all activities happening during diagnosis and intervention were occurring simultaneously. Furthermore, the median time from birth to intervention, and the median time from birth to confirmation of diagnosis, were both more than two times faster for CAH cases than non-CAH cases. It should be noted that all non-CAH cases are inclusive of time-critical and non-time-critical disorders, and have differing denominators based on data entered in the NewSTEPs data repository. This is consistent with state profile data findings, suggesting that NBS programs may prioritize running tests and reporting results for time-critical disorders.

The analysis of the CAH case data submitted by 13 NBS programs for all three years shows that the median time interval of birth to the confirmation of diagnosis was the same compared to that of all CAH cases entered. This indicates that there is not a significant difference in time to diagnosis between the 13 programs that entered data for all three years versus programs did that not enter diagnosis information for all three years.

5. Conclusions

US NBS programs differ in hours of operation, as well as in follow-up definitions and procedures, however the screening methodologies and equipment used for CAH NBS are similar across the US. Furthermore, while there is variability in NBS systems across the US, NewSTEPs facilitates harmonization, and coordinates efforts amongst programs through national data collection, data analysis and technical assistance in order to improve the NBS system.

NewSTEPs' public health surveillance case definitions allow for consistent categorization of newborns at risk of developing an NBS condition. However, there is a lack of data being entered for the diagnostic workup section in the NewSTEPs data repository, making it difficult to apply NewSTEPs case definitions to data. For those programs that have entered data, it is often incomplete, with missing fields. There is a need for better quality CAH-confirmed case data. NewSTEPs continues to encourage NBS programs to provide more complete data, in order to be able to ask questions of datasets and accurately answer those questions.

Although there is room for improvement, the 35 contributing NBS programs fall within the national timeliness recommendations for specimen collection and the reporting of out-of-range results for CAH as a time-critical disorder. This is vital to ensuring that newborns at risk of CAH are appropriately seen by a medical provider in a timely manner. NewSTEPs supports NBS programs in improving timeliness by providing essential tools and techniques needed to successfully implement quality improvement initiatives and champion a quality improvement culture. These tools include national webinars archived on the NewSTEPs' comprehensive resource center, data support and visualization to track improvement, funding opportunities to support initiatives, as well as online forums, training and customized coaching. NewSTEPs will continue to give feedback and data back to NBS programs, and support them in being more analytical towards their screening outcomes. This NewSTEPs model can serve as an example for NBS quality improvement practices worldwide.

Despite data entry challenges, NewSTEPs is committed to increasing the quantity and quality of case definition data in the repository, and will continue to do so via targeted outreach and pursuit of automated data entry options. It is vital for NBS programs to close the case loop with providers and get data back at the public health level, so as to adequately track and monitor newborns at the local, regional and national levels.

Supplementary Materials: Supplementary materials can be found at http://www.mdpi.com/2409-515X/6/3/64/s1.

Author Contributions: Conceptualization, C.Y., S.E., H.D. and T.P.; Data curation, T.P., S.E.; Formal Analysis, H.D.; Visualization, H.D.; Writing—original draft, S.E., H.D.; Writing—review and editing, C.Y., T.P., S.E., H.D and J.O.; Funding acquisition, J.O. All authors have read and agreed to the published version of this manuscript.

Funding: This project is supported by the Health Resources and Services Administration (HRSA) under cooperative agreement #U22MC24078. Its contents are solely the responsibility of the authors and should not be construed as the official position or policy of, nor should any endorsements be inferred by HRSA, HHS, or the US Government.

Conflicts of Interest: The authors declare no conflict of interest.

References

1. NewSTEPs 2019 Annual Report. Available online: https://www.newsteps.org/sites/default/files/nbs-newsteps-2019-annual-report.pdf (accessed on 5 May 2020).
2. Merke, D.; Kabbani, M. Congenital adrenal hyperplasia: Epidemiology, management and practical drug treatment. *Pediatr. Drugs* **2001**, *3*, 599–611. [CrossRef] [PubMed]
3. White, P. Neonatal screening for congenital adrenal hyperplasia. *Nat. Rev. Endocrinol.* **2009**, *5*, 490–498. [CrossRef] [PubMed]
4. NewSTEPs. Available online: https://www.newsteps.org/ (accessed on 5 May 2020).
5. Ojodu, J.; Singh, S.; Kellar-Guenther, Y.; Yusuf, C.; Jones, E.; Wood, T.; Baker, M.; Sontag, M.K. NewSTEPs: The Establishment of a National Newborn Screening Technical Assistance Resource Center. *Int. J. Neonatal Screen.* **2018**, *4*, 1. [CrossRef]
6. NewSTEPs Data Repository User Guide. Available online: https://www.newsteps.org/sites/default/files/newsteps_general_user_guide_june2018_se.pdf (accessed on 5 May 2020).
7. Sontag, M.K.; Sarkar, D.; Comeau, A.M.; Hassell, K.; Botto, L.D.; Parad, R.; Rose, S.R.; Wintergerst, K.A.; Smith-Whitley, K.; Singh, S.; et al. Case Definitions for Conditions Identified by Newborn Screening Public Health Surveillance. *Int. J. Neonatal Screen.* **2018**, *4*, 16. [CrossRef] [PubMed]
8. *Newborn Screening Follow-up; Approved Guideline—Second Edition*; CLSI document NBS02-A2; Clinical and Laboratory Standards Institute: Wayne, PA, USA, 2013.
9. NewSTEPs List of Time-critical Disorders. Available online: https://www.newsteps.org/sites/default/files/case-definitions/qi_source_document_time_critical_disorders_0.pdf (accessed on 5 May 2020).
10. Definition of Term Pregnancy. Available online: https://www.acog.org/clinical/clinical-guidance/committee-opinion/articles/2013/11/definition-of-term-pregnancy (accessed on 8 July 2020).
11. Health Resources and Services Administration Federal Advisory Committees: Newborn Screening Timeliness Goals. Available online: https://www.hrsa.gov/advisory-committees/heritable-disorders/newborn-screening-timeliness.html (accessed on 21 May 2020).
12. NewSTEPs Quality Indicator Source Document. Available online: https://www.newsteps.org/sites/default/files/quality-indicators/quality_indicator_source_document_july_17_2018_se.pdf (accessed on 5 May 2020).
13. NewSTEPs Definitions for Medical Intervention and Diagnosis by Disorder. Available online: https://www.newsteps.org/sites/default/files/case-definitions/case_definition_overview_summary_feb62017.pdf (accessed on 5 May 2020).
14. Held, P.K.; Shapira, S.K.; Hinton, C.F.; Jones, E.; Hannon, W.H.; Ojodu, J. Congenital adrenal hyperplasia cases identified by newborn screening in one- and two-screen states. *Mol. Genet. Metab.* **2015**, *116*, 133–138. [CrossRef] [PubMed]

15. Sontag, M.K.; Miller, J.I.; McKasson, S.; Sheller, R.; Edelman, S.; Yusuf, C.; Singh, S.; Sarkar, D.; Bocchini, J.; Scott, J.; et al. Newborn screening timeliness quality improvement initiative: Impact of national recommendations and data repository. *PLoS ONE* **2020**, *15*, e0231050. [CrossRef] [PubMed]
16. New, M.; Yau, M.; Lekarev, O.; Lin-Su, K.; Parsa, A.; Pina, C.; Yuen, T.; Khattab, A. Congenital Adrenal Hyperplasia. In *Endotext*; Feingold, K.R., Anawalt, B., Boyce, A., Chrousos, G., Dungan, K., Grossman, A., Hershman, J.M., Kaltsas, G., Koch, C., Kopp, P., et al., Eds.; MDText.com, Inc.: South Dartmouth, MA, USA, 2000. Available online: https://www.ncbi.nlm.nih.gov/books/NBK278953/ (accessed on 15 March 2017).
17. Speiser, P.W.; Chawla, R.; Chen, M.; Diaz-Thomas, A.; Finlayson, C.; Rutter, M.M.; Sandberg, D.E.; Shimy, K.; Talib, R.; Cerise, J.; et al. Newborn Screening Protocols and Positive Predictive Value for Congenital Adrenal Hyperplasia Vary across the United States. *Int. J. Neonatal Screen.* **2020**, *6*, 37. [CrossRef]
18. NewSTEPs Case Definitions for Newborn Screening. Available online: https://www.newsteps.org/sites/default/files/case-definitions/classificationtablesmaster_12.13.19_se.pdf (accessed on 5 May 2020).
19. van der Kamp, H.J.; Oudshoorn, C.G.M.; Elvers, B.H.; van Baarle, M.; Otten, B.J.; Wit, J.M.; Verkerk, P.H. Cutoff Levels of 17-α-Hydroxyprogesterone in Neonatal Screening for Congenital Adrenal Hyperplasia Should Be Based on Gestational Age Rather Than on Birth Weight. *J. Clin. Endocrinol. Metab.* **2005**, *90*, 3904–3907. [CrossRef] [PubMed]

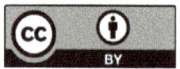

© 2020 by the authors. Licensee MDPI, Basel, Switzerland. This article is an open access article distributed under the terms and conditions of the Creative Commons Attribution (CC BY) license (http://creativecommons.org/licenses/by/4.0/).

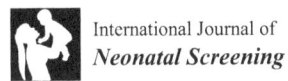

International Journal of
Neonatal Screening

Article

Newborn Screening Protocols and Positive Predictive Value for Congenital Adrenal Hyperplasia Vary across the United States

Phyllis W. Speiser [1,*], Reeti Chawla [2], Ming Chen [3], Alicia Diaz-Thomas [4], Courtney Finlayson [5], Meilan M. Rutter [6], David E. Sandberg [7], Kim Shimy [8], Rashida Talib [1], Jane Cerise [9], Eric Vilain [10], Emmanuèle C. Délot [10] and on behalf of the Disorders/Differences of Sex Development-Translational Research Network (DSD-TRN)

1. Division of Endocrinology, Cohen Children's Medical Ctr of New York, Feinstein Institute for Medical Research, Zucker School of Medicine at Hofstra University, New Hyde Park, NY 11040, USA; rtalib@northwell.edu
2. Division of Endocrinology, Phoenix Children's Hospital, Phoenix, AZ 85016, USA; rchawla@phoenixchildrens.com
3. Division of Endocrinology, CS Mott Children's Hospital, University of Michigan, Ann Arbor, MI 48109, USA; chenming@med.umich.edu
4. Division of Endocrinology, LeBonheur Children's Hospital, University of Tennessee Health Science Center, Memphis, TN 18103, USA; adiaztho@uthsc.edu
5. Division of Endocrinology, Ann & Robert H. Lurie Children's Hospital of Chicago, Northwestern University Feinberg School of Medicine, Chicago, IL 60611, USA; cfinlayson@luriechildrens.org
6. Division of Endocrinology, Cincinnati Children's Hospital Medical Center, University of Cincinnati, Cincinnati, OH 45229, USA; meilan.rutter@cchmc.org
7. Susan B. Meister Child Health Evaluation and Research Center, University of Michigan, Ann Arbor, MI 48109, USA; dsandber@med.umich.edu
8. Division of Endocrinology, Children's National Medical Center, Washington, DC 20010, USA; kim.shimy@childrensnational.org
9. Feinstein Institute for Medical Research, Northwell Health, Manhasset, NY 11030, USA; jcerise@northwell.edu
10. Children's National Hospital, Children's Research Institute and George Washington University, Washington, DC 20010, USA; evilain@gwu.edu (E.V.); edelot@cnmc.org (E.C.D.)
* Correspondence: pspeiser@northwell.edu

Received: 31 March 2020; Accepted: 6 May 2020; Published: 8 May 2020

Abstract: Newborn screening for congenital adrenal hyperplasia (CAH) caused by 21-hydroxylase deficiency is mandated throughout the US. Filter paper blood specimens are assayed for 17-hydroxyprogesterone (17OHP). Prematurity, low birth weight, or critical illness cause falsely elevated results. The purpose of this report is to highlight differences in protocols among US state laboratories. We circulated a survey to state laboratory directors requesting qualitative and quantitative information about individual screening programs. Qualitative and quantitative information provided by 17 state programs were available for analysis. Disease prevalence ranged from 1:9941 to 1:28,661 live births. Four state laboratories mandated a second screen regardless of the initial screening results; most others did so for infants in intensive care units. All but one program utilized birthweight cut-points, but cutoffs varied widely: 17OHP values of 25 to 75 ng/mL for birthweights >2250–2500 g. The positive predictive values for normal birthweight infants varied from 0.7% to 50%, with the highest predictive values based in two of the states with a mandatory second screen. Data were unavailable for negative predictive values. These data imply differences in sensitivity and specificity in CAH screening in the US. Standardization of newborn screening protocols could improve the positive predictive value.

Keywords: adrenal hyperplasia; congenital; newborn screening; standardization

1. Introduction

Newborn screening for congenital adrenal hyperplasia caused by steroid 21-hydroxylase deficiency (CAH-21) is mandated in the United States, 35 other countries, and in portions of 17 additional countries. Most of the US states report participation of 99.9% or higher [1]. The rationale for screening is to recognize and promptly treat the potentially life-threatening severe salt-wasting classic form of CAH. The overall prevalence of classic CAH-21 is approximately 1:14,000 to 1:18,000, of whom 75% have the salt-wasting form and 25% have non-salt-wasting or so-called simple virilizing CAH (summarized in [2]). Case fatality rates (lethality) of ~4% have been estimated for the era prior to newborn screening, presumably due to salt-wasting adrenal crisis, less frequent in the era of screening [3]. Affected 46,XY males cannot readily be identified without screening, as external genital virilization will flag the diagnosis only in 46,XX individuals. Lethality estimates were based on a rising disease prevalence, increased male to female case ratios, and increased salt wasting to simple virilizing case ratios observed since the advent of screening in the 1980s [4–6]. Other benefits of screening, aside from reduced infant mortality, have included less severe hyponatremia, shorter hospitalizations for infants identified with CAH [7–10], fewer learning disabilities as sequelae of salt-wasting crises [11,12], fewer reports of regret in the assigned gender of rearing [13,14], and potentially better growth outcomes [15]. Newborn screening protocols for measuring the typical marker steroid, 17-hydroxyprogesterone (17OHP), cut-points for abnormal values, and reporting of results are not standardized. Instead, each state develops and adapts its own procedures. The purpose of this report is to describe the varied CAH-21 screening practices in the US based on a sampling of individual state programs.

2. Materials and Methods

Pediatric endocrinologists and other members of the Disorders/Differences of Sex Development Translational Research Network (DSD-TRN) circulated a survey (Supplementary Data) to state laboratory directors of their own states and neighboring state programs requesting qualitative and quantitative information about CAH screening programs. Questions included basic epidemiologic statistics for the number of infants screened, number of positive screens, and number of cases confirmed as CAH. Details of the assay methods, cut-points, and factors considered for stratifying abnormal values were queried. We asked about the personnel responsible for reporting and receiving abnormal results for hospitalized and discharged infants, and criteria for follow-up testing. Data sets were returned from 17 states, and descriptive statistics were analyzed for the calendar year 2017. Results shown refer to those obtained in normal birthweight infants. Confirmed CAH cases (true positives) were defined as those reported to the state screening programs as meeting standard confirmatory diagnostic criteria for classic CAH, including a baseline serum 17OHP >10,000 ng/dL (or 300 nmol/L), cosyntropin testing resulting in markedly elevated stimulated serum 17OHP [16], and/or *CYP21A2* genotyping indicating known classic disease-causing mutations. False positives included those infants with 17OHP results above the cut-off point for birthweight but ultimately confirmed as not having CAH. Some of these data were presented in spring 2019 at The Endocrine Society Meeting, New Orleans, LA, USA and at the National Newborn Screening Board Meeting, Bethesda, MD, USA.

Statistical Methods

The reported number of screens, number of positive screens (excluding low birth weight infants), and number of endocrinologist-confirmed CAH cases from 2017 were used to estimate the number of true negative cases, prevalence, and positive predictive value (PPV). We arbitrarily assumed no false negative results for all programs, as negative screens were not referred for definitive diagnosis, and their final status was not reported to the state laboratories. Therefore, the number of confirmed cases was estimated for each state as the number of positive screens who were confirmed as having

CAH, and the number of true negative cases was estimated for each state as the total number screened minus the sum of true positive and false positive cases. Under the assumption of no false negatives, the estimate of the number of confirmed cases served as a lower bound on the number of confirmed cases, and the estimate of the number of true negative cases served as an upper bound on the number of true negative cases. In other words, if there were any false negatives, this would result in a higher number of confirmed cases and a lower number of true negative cases. Similarly, the prevalence, estimated for each state as the number of confirmed positives divided by the total number screened, was a lower bound estimate. PPV for each state was estimated as 100 times the number of confirmed cases divided by the number of positive screens. The weighted mean prevalence was calculated as the sum of the prevalence for each state weighted by the proportion of patients screened for that state out of all 17 states. Under the assumption of no false negatives, because all newborns are screened, this is equal to the sum of all states' confirmed cases divided by the sum of infants screened in all states.

Spearman correlation coefficients (shown as r_s below) were calculated between PPV and the 17OHP cut-off point, and between PPV and prevalence.

A p-value < 0.05 was considered statistically significant. All analyses were conducted using SAS version 9.4 (SAS Institute Inc., Cary, NC, USA). Figure 1 was created using the package ggplot2 in R version 3.6.1.

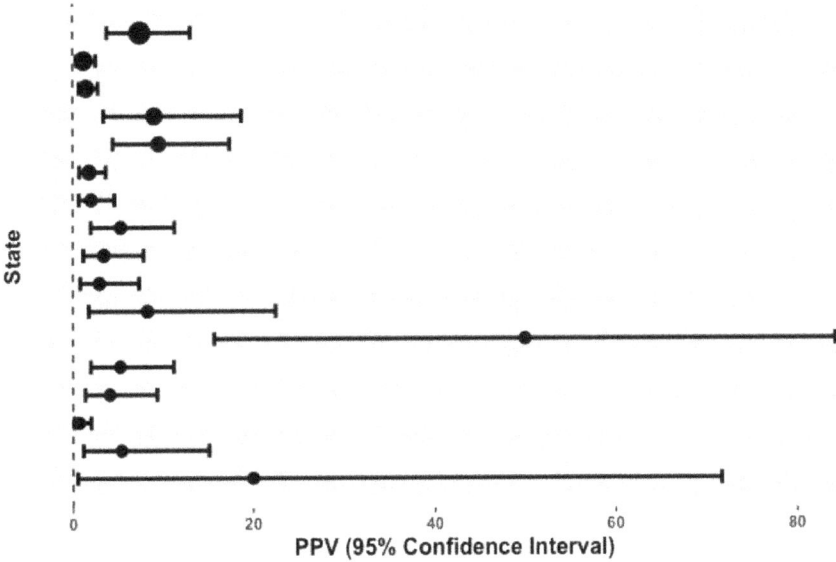

Figure 1. The positive predictive values (PPVs) calculated for each state are shown, with their respective 95% confidence intervals. States are ordered from the smallest to largest number of screens performed (from bottom up on y axis). Dot size is related to the number of screens performed (numerical data used are shown in Table 1).

Table 1. CAH newborn screening by state.

#Screened (Total = 1,564,756)	#Referred Positive (Total = 3217)	#Confirmed CAH (Total = 93)	Prevalence (Weighted Mean = 1:16,825)	PPV (95% CI) IQR = [2.02 to 8.33]	Birth Weight Cut-Off Point (Grams)	17OHP Cut-Off Point (ng/mL) (Mean = 41.2)	Two-Screens Mandate
230,431	146	11	1:20,948	7.53 (3.82–13.08)	>2251	35	N
171,964	506	6	1:28,661	1.19 (0.44–2.56)	>2500	55	N
138,226	608	9	1:15,358	1.48 (0.68–2.79)	>2500	70	N
135,590	66	6	1:22,598	9.09 (3.41–18.74)	>2500	30	N
109,740	94	9	1:12,193	9.57 (4.47–17.4)	>2500	65	N
104,000	387	7	1:14,857	1.81 (0.73–3.69)	>2250	25	N
84,000	247	5	1:16,800	2.02 (0.66–4.66)	>2500	30	N
81,117	112	6	1:13,520	5.36 (1.99–11.30)	>2500	50	Y
79,948	144	5	1:15,990	3.47 (1.14–7.92)	>2249	37	N
79,000	135	4	1:19,750	2.96 (0.81–7.41)	≥2500	35	Y
72,440	36	3	1:24,147	8.33 (1.75–22.47)	>2251	75	N
61,500	8	4	1:15,375	50.00 (15.70–84.30)	>2500	25	Y
59,643	113	6	1:9941	5.31 (1.97–11.2)	No values given		N
55,935	121	5	1:11,187	4.13 (1.36–9.38)	>2500	25	N
53,361	434	3	1:17,787	0.69 (0.14–2.01)	>2500	30	N
36,361	55	3	1:12,120	5.45 (1.14–15.12)	≥2500	38.3	N
11,500	5	1	1:11,500	20.00 (0.51–71.64)	≥2300	35	Y

3. Results

3.1. Epidemiology

Completed questionnaires were provided by 17 states and were analyzed (Table 1). Partial responses from 3 additional states were not included. The single largest state screening population in our survey included >230,000 infants in a single year, and the smallest only 11,500. More cases were referred for follow-up and confirmatory testing, and then were verified as having CAH. States mandating a second screening sample referred only those second positive screens. In this survey, there were a total of 93 confirmed cases. The prevalence of CAH ranged from 1:9941 to 1:28,661 live births, with a weighted mean prevalence of 1:16,825, similar to published estimates (Table 1). We were unable to obtain mortality or morbidity statistics specific to CAH.

3.2. Assays and Cut-Off Points

All laboratories used fluoroimmunoassay for 17OHP measurement in filter paper blood samples (DELFIA time-resolved fluorescence assay, Perkin Elmer, Waltham, MA, USA) obtained after 24 h of life. Most states performed the assay in their own laboratories, while some sent the samples to Perkin Elmer's facilities using the same assay kits. All but one of the programs utilized birthweight cut-points, but cutoffs varied widely, from 17OHP values of 25 to 75 ng/mL (mean 41.2 ng/mL) for normal birthweights >2250–2500 g (Table 1). Cut-off points for lower birth weights were generally higher. Four state laboratories in our survey mandated a second screen regardless of initial screening results, and results of the second screen were used in this analysis where available. Most states utilized a later or second screen for infants in intensive care units, as early screening of sick, premature, or low birth weight infants gives many false positive results, contributing to lower positive predictive values [2].

The estimated positive predictive values for normal birthweight infants varied from 0.7% to 50% (mean 8.1%; median 5.3%). No statistically significant correlation was observed between PPV and the 17OHP cut-off point ($r_s = -0.0059$, $p = 0.98$, $n = 16$), nor between PPV and prevalence ($r_s = 0.21$, $p = 0.42$, $n = 17$). The highest predictive values were found in two of the four states with a mandatory second screen, with estimated PPV values greater than 1.5 times the interquartile range of 6.3. (Table 1, Figure 1).

3.3. Post-Analytical Procedures

There were no data concerning the cross-validation of assays carried out in different state laboratories. Each state reported positive results differently. Methods included phone calls, faxed documents, and/or mailed letters. Reporting went to a variety of reportees, including administrative aides, nurses, genetic counselors, or pediatric endocrinologists. Reports on infants with mildly or moderately abnormal screens who had been discharged from the birth hospital typically were sent to the primary care pediatrician listed on the hospital discharge. Information was not available regarding the content of counseling to the families. Infants with borderline or mildly elevated results usually underwent repeat screening. When an abnormal screen was obtained for a hospitalized infant, the neonatologist was informed, and a repeat sample obtained shortly thereafter. Those with more markedly abnormal results were most often referred directly to the pediatric endocrinologist at the state-designated center and underwent further confirmatory tests, such as a cosyntropin stimulation test if indicated, at the clinician's discretion. We were unable to obtain data on the exact time between the reporting of results to the clinician and the start of treatment, as such data were not collected by the state laboratories. There was no consistent means of reporting infants missed by screening who later proved to be affected with classic CAH, and thus data were unavailable for false negative results or negative predictive values. Moreover, limited or no phenotypic data were recorded by state laboratories about the infants' genital examination or other clinical features; no long-term outcomes were collected. Thus, we could not ascertain whether screening contributed to the prevention of salt wasting, nor were we able to distinguish salt-wasting from non-salt-wasting types of CAH.

4. Discussion

The primary aim of this report was to document differences in CAH newborn screening protocols. Our survey of about one-third of the US states confirms that screening for CAH using a single sample primary fluoroimmunoassay for 17OHP is associated with low positive predictive values [17]. In this report, we only included data related to the positive predictive value for normal birthweight infants, as prematurity, low birthweight, and sampling within the first 24 h of life are major causes of false positive results (reviewed in [2]). Although all laboratories used the same fluoroimmunoassay kit, conditions in the individual laboratories may have contributed to the lack of correlation between the cut-off point and positive predictive value. Cross-validation of assays might reduce some of the variability. Alternatively, these observations may be due to the relatively small number of confirmed positive cases in each state sample.

Protocols for CAH newborn screening have been adapted and implemented separately by each state laboratory in the US over the past several decades. Publications have generally reported data unique to an individual state screening program with a few exceptions [18,19]. For instance, at present, 13 states mandate a second screen at about two weeks of life in part due to the relatively low positive predictive value of the initial screen. These programs tend to show a higher disease prevalence compared with those only performing a single screen [18]. However, those later diagnosed infants are often non-salt-wasting, which some argue is not the objective of screening. In this survey, we could not ascertain whether screening contributed to the prevention of salt wasting, nor were we able to distinguish salt-wasting from non-salt-wasting types of CAH. According to the current Endocrine Society CAH Guidelines [2], all infants detected with CAH in the newborn period are to be treated with a combination of glucocorticoids, mineralocorticoid, and sodium chloride supplements. Thus, most pediatric endocrinologists no longer wait until evidence of salt wasting is observed before starting the patient on these standard treatments.

Alternative diagnostic methods and screening protocols have previously been evaluated. Suggestions for quality improvement include gestational age-based cut-off points [5,20] or a combination of birthweight and gestational age [21]. Implementation of a second screen at two weeks of life improves the positive predictive value as noted but adds cost and may be impractical or logistically difficult in some regions. A second tier test, specifically liquid chromatography-tandem mass spectrometry (LC-MS/MS), has been cited as a useful adjunctive test [22,23] that may be adapted to measure an extended steroid profile [24], although it is not currently suitable for high-volume screening at the first tier due to time constraints. At present, genotyping *CYP21A2* is not utilized in most US programs for either primary or secondary screening due to the complexity of test interpretation, time constraints, and costs [2], although this may change in the future.

Quality improvement efforts should be directed at enhanced communication between clinicians and state laboratories and transparent reporting of states' efforts on a national platform. This would include not only the creation of common disease screening panels but also the standardization of protocols, with the aim of eventually achieving a uniform set of best practices [25,26]. With respect to the negative predictive value of screening, a centralized registry of CAH cases diagnosed after the newborn period would aid in capturing false negative tests from the newborn period. Colorado published data citing a 28% false negative rate in the primary screen once a second screen was implemented [27]. New York reported only three false negative cases from their single screen over a span of 7 years, but this is highly dependent on complete follow-up and physician reporting [19]. Surprisingly, Minnesota found a 32% false negative rate, even in the context of two screens [28]. The causes of such disparities are unclear and should be investigated. Finally, there are negative psychological implications to conveying inaccurate screening results to parents, and improving these protocols could have important mental health ramifications. Nationwide (NewSteps [29] and the Disorders/Differences of

Sex Development-Translational Research Network (DSD-TRN). [30,31]) and international (Clinical and Laboratory Standards Institute [32]) collaboratives offer opportunities to explore and compare screening outcomes and develop best practices.

Supplementary Materials: Supplementary materials can be found at http://www.mdpi.com/2409-515X/6/2/37/s1.

Author Contributions: Conceptualization, P.W.S., A.D.-T., C.F. and M.M.R.; Data curation, P.W.S., M.C., A.D.-T., C.F., M.M.R., K.S. and R.T.; Formal analysis, P.W.S., R.T. and J.C.; Funding acquisition, D.E.S., E.V. and E.C.D.; Investigation, P.W.S., R.C. and E.C.D.; Methodology, R.T. and J.C.; Project administration, D.E.S., E.V. and E.C.D.; Supervision, P.W.S.; Writing—original draft, P.W.S.; Writing—review & editing, P.W.S., R.C., M.C., A.D.-T., C.F., M.R., D.E.S., K.S., R.T., J.C., E.V. and E.C.D. All authors have read and agreed to the published version of the manuscript.

Funding: This research was funded by NIH-NICHD 1R01 HD093450, DSD-Translational Research Network.

Acknowledgments: We thank state newborn screening laboratory personnel for their cooperation.

Conflicts of Interest: The authors declare no conflict of interest.

Abbreviations

CAH	Congenital adrenal hyperplasia
CAH-21	CAH due to steroid 21-hydroxylase deficiency
17OHP	17-hydroxyprogesterone
DSD-TRN	Disorders/Differences of Sex Development Translational Research Network
PPV	Positive predictive value
IQR	Interquartile range
LC-MS/MS	Liquid chromatography-tandem mass spectrometry

References

1. Eunice Kennedy Shriver National Institute of Child Health and Human Development. Available online: https://www.nichd.nih.gov/health/topics/newborn/conditioninfo/infants-screened (accessed on 22 April 2020).
2. Speiser, P.W.; Arlt, W.; Auchus, R.J.; Baskin, L.S.; Conway, G.S.; Merke, D.P.; Meyer-Bahlburg, H.F.L.; Miller, W.L.; Murad, M.H.; Oberfield, S.E.; et al. Congenital Adrenal Hyperplasia Due to Steroid 21-Hydroxylase Deficiency: An Endocrine Society Clinical Practice Guideline. *J. Clin. Endocrinol. Metab.* **2018**, *103*, 4043–4088. [CrossRef]
3. Gidlof, S.; Wedell, A.; Guthenberg, C.; von, D.U.; Nordenstrom, A. Nationwide neonatal screening for congenital adrenal hyperplasia in sweden: A 26-year longitudinal prospective population-based study. *JAMA Pediatr.* **2014**, *168*, 567–574. [CrossRef]
4. Gidlof, S.; Falhammar, H.; Thilen, A.; von, D.U.; Ritzen, M.; Wedell, A.; Nordenstrom, A. One hundred years of congenital adrenal hyperplasia in Sweden: A retrospective, population-based cohort study. *Lancet Diabetes Endocrinol.* **2013**, *1*, 35–42. [CrossRef]
5. van der Linde, A.A.A.; Schönbeck, Y.; van der Kamp, H.J.; van den Akker, E.L.T.; van Albada, M.E.; Boelen, A.; Finken, M.J.J.; Hannema, S.E.; Hoorweg-Nijman, G.; Odink, R.J.; et al. Evaluation of the Dutch neonatal screening for congenital adrenal hyperplasia. *Arch. Dis. Child* **2019**, *104*, 653–657. [CrossRef] [PubMed]
6. Guran, T.; Tezel, B.; Gurbuz, F.; Selver Eklioglu, B.; Hatipoglu, N.; Kara, C.; Simsek, E.; Cizmecioglu, F.; Ozon, A.; Bas, F.; et al. Neonatal screening for congenital adrenal hyperplasia in Turkey: A pilot study with 38,935 infants. *J. Clin. Res. Pediatr. Endocrinol.* **2019**, *11*, 13–23. [CrossRef] [PubMed]
7. Brosnan, P.G.; Brosnan, C.A.; Kemp, S.F.; Domek, D.B.; Jelley, D.H.; Blackett, P.R.; Riley, W.J. Effect of Newborn Screening for Congenital Adrenal Hyperplasia. *Arch. Pediatr. Adolesc. Med.* **1999**, *153*, 1272. [CrossRef] [PubMed]
8. Thilen, A.; Nordenstrom, A.; Hagenfeldt, L.; von Dobeln, U.; Guthenberg, C.; Larsson, A. Benefits of Neonatal Screening for Congenital Adrenal Hyperplasia (21-Hydroxylase Deficiency) in Sweden. *Pediatrics* **1998**, *101*, e11. [CrossRef] [PubMed]
9. Van der Kamp, H.J.; Noordam, K.; Elvers, B.; Van Baarle, M.; Otten, B.J.; Verkerk, P.H. Newborn screening for congenital adrenal hyperplasia in the Netherlands. *Pediatrics* **2001**, *108*, 1320–1324. [CrossRef] [PubMed]

10. Morikawa, S.; Nakamura, A.; Fujikura, K.; Fukushi, M.; Hotsubo, T.; Miyata, J.; Ishizu, K.; Tajima, T. Results from 28 years of newborn screening for congenital adrenal hyperplasia in sapporo. *Clin. Pediatr. Endocrinol.* **2014**, *23*, 35–43. [CrossRef]
11. Nass, R.; Baker, S. Learning disabilities in children with congenital adrenal hyperplasia. *J. Child Neurol.* **1991**, *6*, 306–312. [CrossRef]
12. Inozemtseva, O.; Matute, E.; Juárez, J. Learning disabilities spectrum and sexual dimorphic abilities in girls with congenital adrenal hyperplasia. *J. Child Neurol.* **2008**, *23*, 862–869. [CrossRef] [PubMed]
13. Lee, P.A.; Witchel, S.F. 46,XX patients with congenital adrenal hyperplasia: Initial assignment as male, reassigned female. *J. Pediatr. Endocrinol. Metab.* **2005**, *18*, 125–132. [CrossRef] [PubMed]
14. Apóstolos, R.A.C.; Canguçu-Campinho, A.K.; Lago, R.; Costa, A.C.S.; Oliveira, L.M.B.; Toralles, M.B.; Barroso, U. Gender Identity and Sexual Function in 46,XX Patients with Congenital Adrenal Hyperplasia Raised as Males. *Arch. Sex. Behav.* **2018**, *47*, 2491–2496. [CrossRef] [PubMed]
15. Muthusamy, K.; Elamin, M.B.; Smushkin, G.; Murad, M.H.; Lampropulos, J.F.; Elamin, K.B.; Abu Elnour, N.O.; Gallegos-Orozco, J.F.; Fatourechi, M.M.; Agrwal, N.; et al. Clinical review: Adult height in patients with congenital adrenal hyperplasia: A systematic review and metaanalysis. *J. Clin. Endocrinol. Metab.* **2010**, *95*, 4161–4172. [CrossRef]
16. Wilson, R.C.; Mercado, A.B.; Cheng, K.C.; New, M.I. Steroid 21-hydroxylase deficiency: Genotype may not predict phenotype. *J. Clin. Endocrinol. Metab.* **1995**, *80*, 2322–2329.
17. White, P.C. Optimizing newborn screening for congenital adrenal hyperplasia. *J. Pediatr.* **2013**, *163*, 10–12. [CrossRef]
18. Held, P.K.; Shapira, S.K.; Hinton, C.F.; Jones, E.; Hannon, W.H.; Ojodu, J. Congenital adrenal hyperplasia cases identified by newborn screening in one- and two-screen states. *Mol. Genet. Metab.* **2015**, *116*, 133–138. [CrossRef]
19. Pearce, M.; DeMartino, L.; McMahon, R.; Hamel, R.; Maloney, B.; Stansfield, D.M.; McGrath, E.C.; Occhionero, A.; Gearhart, A.; Caggana, M.; et al. Newborn screening for congenital adrenal hyperplasia in New York State. *Mol. Genet. Metab. Rep.* **2016**, *7*, 1–7. [CrossRef]
20. Tsuji, A.; Konishi, K.; Hasegawa, S.; Anazawa, A.; Onishi, T.; Ono, M.; Morio, T.; Kitagawa, T.; Kashimada, K. Newborn screening for congenital adrenal hyperplasia in Tokyo, Japan from 1989 to 2013: A retrospective population-based study. *BMC Pediatr.* **2015**, *15*, 209. [CrossRef]
21. Pode-Shakked, N.; Blau, A.; Pode-Shakked, B.; Tiosano, D.; Weintrob, N.; Eyal, O.; Zung, A.; Levy-Khademi, F.; Tenenbaum-Rakover, Y.; Zangen, D.; et al. Combined gestational age- and birth weight-adjusted cutoffs for newborn screening of congenital adrenal hyperplasia. *J. Clin. Endocrinol. Metab.* **2019**, *104*, 3172–3180. [CrossRef]
22. Monostori, P.; Szabo, P.; Marginean, O.; Bereczki, C.; Karg, E. Concurrent confirmation and differential diagnosis of congenital adrenal hyperplasia from dried blood spots: Application of a second-tier LC-MS/MS assay in a cross-border cooperation for newborn screening. *Horm. Res. Paediatr.* **2015**, *84*, 311–318. [CrossRef] [PubMed]
23. Gaudl, A.; Kratzsch, J.; Ceglarek, U. Advancement in steroid hormone analysis by LC-MS/MS in clinical routine diagnostics-A three year recap from serum cortisol to dried blood 17α-hydroxyprogesterone. *J. Steroid Biochem. Mol. Biol.* **2019**, *192*, 105389. [CrossRef] [PubMed]
24. Bialk, E.; Lasarev, M.R.; Held, P.K. Wisconsin's screening algorithm for the identification of newborns with congenital adrenal hyperplasia. *Int. J. Neonatal Screen.* **2019**, *5*, 33. [CrossRef]
25. Martínez-Morillo, E.; Prieto García, B.; Álvarez Menéndez, F.V. Challenges for Worldwide Harmonization of Newborn Screening Programs. *Clin. Chem.* **2016**, *62*, 689–698. [CrossRef] [PubMed]
26. Lloyd-Puryear, M.; Brower, A.; Berry, S.A.; Brosco, J.P.; Bowdish, B.; Watson, M.S. Foundation of the Newborn Screening Translational Research Network and its tools for research. *Genet. Med.* **2019**, *21*, 1271–1279. [CrossRef] [PubMed]
27. Chan, C.L.; McFann, K.; Taylor, L.; Wright, D.; Zeitler, P.S.; Barker, J.M. Congenital adrenal hyperplasia and the second newborn screen. *J. Pediatr.* **2013**, *163*, 109–113.e101. [CrossRef] [PubMed]
28. Sarafoglou, K.; Banks, K.; Gaviglio, A.; Hietala, A.; McCann, M.; Thomas, W. Comparison of one-tier and two-tier newborn screening metrics for congenital adrenal hyperplasia. *Pediatrics* **2012**, *130*, e1261–e1268. [CrossRef]

29. Glidewell, J.; Grosse, S.D.; Riehle-Colarusso, T.; Pinto, N.; Hudson, J.; Daskalov, R.; Gaviglio, A.; Darby, E.; Singh, S.; Sontag, M. Actions in Support of Newborn Screening for Critical Congenital Heart Disease-United States, 2011–2018. *MMWR Morb. Mortal. Wkly. Rep.* **2019**, *68*, 107–111. [CrossRef]
30. Sandberg, D.E.; Gardner, M.; Callens, N.; Mazur, T.; the DSD-TRN Psychosocial Workgroup; the DSD-TRN Advocacy Advisory Network; Accord Alliance. Interdisciplinary care in disorders/differences of sex development (DSD): The psychosocial component of the DSD-Translational research network. *Am. J. Med. Genet. C Semin. Med. Genet.* **2017**, *175*, 279–292. [CrossRef]
31. Délot, E.C.; Papp, J.C.; Sandberg, D.E.; Vilain, E.; Workgroup, D.-T.G. Genetics of Disorders of Sex Development: The DSD-TRN Experience. *Endocrinol. Metab. Clin. N. Am.* **2017**, *46*, 519–537. [CrossRef]
32. *Defining, Establishing, and Verifying Reference Intervals in the Clinical Laboratory; Approved Guidelines-Third Edition CLSI Document (2010)*, 3rd ed.; CLSI: Wayne, PA, USA, 2010; Volume EP28-A3c.

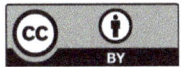

© 2020 by the authors. Licensee MDPI, Basel, Switzerland. This article is an open access article distributed under the terms and conditions of the Creative Commons Attribution (CC BY) license (http://creativecommons.org/licenses/by/4.0/).

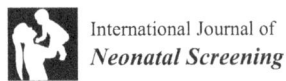

Article

Measurement of 17-Hydroxyprogesterone by LCMSMS Improves Newborn Screening for CAH Due to 21-Hydroxylase Deficiency in New Zealand

Mark R. de Hora [1,*], Natasha L. Heather [1], Tejal Patel [1], Lauren G. Bresnahan [1], Dianne Webster [1] and Paul L. Hofman [2]

[1] Newborn Screening, Specialist Chemical Pathology, LabPlus, Auckland City Hospital, Auckland 1023, New Zealand; NHeather@adhb.govt.nz (N.L.H.); tejalP@adhb.govt.nz (T.P.); lbresnahan@adhb.govt.nz (L.G.B.); diannew@adhb.govt.nz (D.W.)
[2] Clinical Research Unit, Liggins Institute, University of Auckland, Auckland 1010, New Zealand; p.hofman@auckland.ac.nz
* Correspondence: mdehora@adhb.govt.nz

Received: 24 December 2019; Accepted: 24 January 2020; Published: 28 January 2020

Abstract: The positive predictive value of newborn screening for congenital adrenal hyperplasia due to 21-hydroxylase deficiency was <2% in New Zealand. This is despite a bloodspot second-tier immunoassay method for 17-hydroxyprogesterone measurement with an additional solvent extract step to reduce the number of false positive screening tests. We developed a liquid chromatography tandem mass spectrometry (LCMSMS) method to measure 17-hydroxyprogesterone in bloodspots to replace our current second-tier immunoassay method. The method was assessed using reference material and residual samples with a positive newborn screening result. Correlation with the second-tier immunoassay was determined and the method was implemented. Newborn screening performance was assessed by comparing screening metrics 2 years before and 2 years after LCMSMS implementation. Screening data analysis demonstrated the number of false positive screening tests was reduced from 172 to 40 in the 2 years after LCMSMS implementation. The positive predictive value of screening significantly increased from 1.71% to 11.1% (X^2 test, $p < 0.0001$). LCMSMS analysis of 17OHP as a second-tier test significantly improves screening specificity for CAH due to 21-hydroxylase deficiency in New Zealand.

Keywords: congenital adrenal hyperplasia; 17-hydroxyprogesterone; newborn screening; liquid chromatography tandem mass spectrometry

1. Introduction

Congenital adrenal hyperplasia (CAH) represents a group of inherited disorders characterised by absent or reduced adrenal cortisol synthesis. Approximately 90% of CAH is caused by mutations in the CYP21A2 gene resulting in reduced activity of adrenal steroid 21-hydroxylase. 21-Hydroxylase catalyses the conversion of 17α-hydroxyprogesterone (17OHP) to 11-deoxycortisol and progesterone to 11-deoxycorticosterone, the respective precursors to cortisol and aldosterone [1].

Reduced synthesis of aldosterone can lead to life threatening salt wasting, vascular collapse and an Addisonian crisis in the neonatal period. Reduced cortisol synthesis results in a loss of normal feedback to the hypothalamus and pituitary gland leading to an increase in pituitary adrenocorticotrophic hormone (ACTH) release. Increased ACTH levels cause adrenal hyperplasia with increased androgen synthesis and the concomitant rise in intermediate metabolites in the steroidogenesis pathway.

Many countries now perform newborn screening for CAH due to 21-hydroxylase deficiency to prevent life threatening salt-wasting crises and hypoglycaemia in early infancy. The screening test involves measurement of 17OHP by immunoassay in dried blood collected onto specialised blood collection paper [2]. Screening is sensitive for the severe salt-wasting form of CAH but can be confounded by high concentrations of cross reactive 17OHP steroid precursors and their sulphated conjugates, which are present in the first 48 h after birth and longer in pre-term neonates [3]. 17OHP levels may also be elevated due to illness, stress and biological variation [4,5].

In New Zealand, newborn screening specimens with an elevated 17OHP by immunoassay are subjected to a second-tier immunoassay after solvent extraction to remove polar steroids conjugates.

The goal of second-tier testing is to confirm elevated 17OHP levels and thus reduce the number of false positive screening results. The number of falsely elevated results however, remains high as non-polar interfering steroids, such as pregnenolone and 17OH-pregnenolone are not removed by solvent extraction [6]. In 2016, the positive predictive value of CAH screening in New Zealand was estimated at 1.08% [7] meaning that 100 neonates have unnecessary specimen recollections for every case of CAH detected.

Liquid chromatography tandem mass spectrometry (LCMSMS) offers a more analytically specific method of 17OHP measurement as compared with immunoassay. LCMSMS is now sufficiently sensitive for steroid analysis in bloodspots but chromatography is required to separate isobaric steroids and reduce matrix ion suppression. The technique is not suitable for high throughput population screening but is routinely used by screening programmes as a second tier test to confirm positive newborn screening tests or reduce the number of false positives for a range of metabolic disorders [8].

Our goal was to develop a simple and reliable method to measure 17OHP in bloodspots as a second-tier test to reduce the false positive rate of newborn screening for CAH in New Zealand. Correlation between LCMSMS and the immunoassay for 17OHP is reported to be poor in neonates [9] but better in 17OHP bloodspot reference material [10]. Therefore, our approach was to develop a LCMSMS method and determine its performance using 17OHP bloodspot reference material, proficiency testing samples from a quality assurance scheme and bloodspots enriched with 17OHP prepared in our laboratory. We determined the relationship between LCMSMS and immunoassay in 17OHP proficiency testing samples from a certified quality assurance programme and in bloodspots from neonates with false positive and true positive newborn screening results to confirm the suitability of LCMSMS for our screening protocols. We then implemented LCMSMS as a second-tier test and assessed the performance by comparing screening parameters prior to and after LCMSMS implementation.

2. Materials and Methods

2.1. Reagents

17-hydroxyprogesterone and formic acid were purchased from Sigma-Aldrich (Auckland, NZ), d8-hydroxyprogesterone was purchased from SCIVAC (Hornsby, NSW, Australia). 17-hydroxyprenenolone sulphate was purchased from Steraloids (Newport, Rhode Island, USA). LCMSMS grade acetonitrile, methanol, acetone and isopropanol were purchased from Thermo Fisher NZ (Auckland, NZ).

2.2. Calibrators and Controls

Calibrators and control materials were manufactured using donor whole blood with plasma run off (New Zealand Blood Service). Red cells were washed 3 times with saline before 55% haematocrit blood was made using a serum substitute (Serasub, CST Technologies, NY, USA) to replicate neonatal blood. A stock standard steroid solution was made by dissolving 33.1 mg 17OHP in 10 mL ethanol (10 mM 17OHP) and diluting in saline to make a 33.33 µM spiking solution. Bloodspot 17OHP calibrators were made by adding 0, 15 µL, 30 µL, 60 µL, 120 µL and 240 µL of spiking solution to 20 mL aliquots of 55% haematocrit blood to make 6 calibrators ranging from 0 to 400 nmol/L. Three controls were prepared using the same procedure with 10 µL, 45 µL and 90 µL of 17OHP spiking solution. Blood was mixed for 1 h and spotted onto blood collection paper (Whatman 903™), dried at room temperature and stored at −20 °C until analysis.

A stock solution of internal standard was prepared by dissolving 1.25 mg of d_8-17OHP in 500 mL methanol divided into glass vials and stored at −80 °C. A working internal standard (36.9 nmol/L) was prepared by diluting 5 mL stock in 50 mL methanol.

To evaluate the interference of sulphated steroids, 17-hydroxypregnenolone sulphate enriched samples were prepared by adding 240 µL, 120 µL, 60 µL and 30 µL of 333.3 µM solution to 20 mL of 55% haematocrit blood. Blood was mixed for 1 h and spotted onto blood collection paper, dried at room temperature and stored at −20 °C until analysis. The final concentrations of 17-hydroxypregnenolone sulphate were 500, 1000, 2000 and 4000 nmol/L.

2.3. Bloodspot Samples

148 residual newborn screening specimens with out-of-range 17OHP levels (previously used for second-tier immunoassay) were subjected to LCMSMS. Of these, 132 were from infants without CAH (i.e., they had a false positive screen result) and 16 from affected infants.

Certified quality control material (3 levels) enriched with known quantities of 17OHP were used to assess accuracy and recovery. Certified material was supplied by the Centres for Disease Control and Prevention (CDC, Atlanta, USA) Newborn Screening Quality Assurance Scheme.

Control material (3 levels) prepared with the method calibrators were used to assess precision. The interference from sulphated steroid conjugates was assessed using 17-hydroxypregnenolone sulphate enriched bloodspot material.

Thirty three residual external quality assurance samples (EQA) supplied by a CDC Newborn Screening Proficiency Scheme were used to determine the correlation between LCMSMS and immunoassay methods of analysis.

2.4. Immunoassay Protocols of CAH Newborn Screening

Newborn screening specimens are collected from neonates by heel prick onto blood collection cards 48–72 h after birth. In New Zealand, further samples are collected at 2 weeks for babies born with a birthweight (BW) of ≤1500 g and a third sample is collected at 4 weeks if the BW < 1000 g. A screening test is considered positive if a further unscheduled intervention, such as a sample recollect or a clinical referral is warranted.

The primary screening test for CAH due to 21-hydroxylase deficiency is 17OHP measurement carried out using a time resolved fluoroimmunometric direct immunoassay (Perkin Elmer, Turku, Finland). Newborn screening specimens were subjected to an additional immunoassay analysis after solvent extraction when the primary test result was above the newborn screening cut-off. For the extracted immunoassay, a single 3 mm bloodspot, calibrators and controls were punched in 1.5 mL polypropylene tubes. Bloodspots were eluted with 200 µL of 0.1 M phosphate buffer followed by extraction with 1 mL of diethyl ether. Extracts were transferred to glass tubes, dried under nitrogen, reconstituted in immunoassay kit buffer and analysed. Bloodspot calibration material (6 levels) is included in kits by the manufacturer with ranges from approximately 10 nmol/L to 300 nmol/L.

For the primary screening test, 17OHP concentrations by direct immunoassay of ≥37 nmol/L in neonates with a birth-weight (BW) ≤1500 g or ≥27 nmol/L if BW >1500 g were considered out of range and subjected to a second-tier test. The second-tier immunoassay test was considered out of range and screen positive for CAH if the 17OHP concentration was ≥34 nmol/L in neonates with a BW ≤ 1500 g or ≥24 nmol/L in neonates with a BW > 1500 g. A CAH screen is considered positive if further action is required on the baby, i.e., and additional sample or a clinical referral. Hence, an out-of-range result at 48 h on a 1400 g BW baby would not be considered a positive screen as a further sample is scheduled to be taken at 2 weeks.

2.5. Sample Preparation for LCMSMS Method

For the LCMSMS method, 2 × 3 mm (6.4 µL) dried blood spots were added to a 96-deep well polypropylene micro titre plate. 20 µL of internal standard was added to each well followed by 200 µL of 80% acetonitrile in water. Plates were sealed and mixed gently for 1 h on a plate mixer and spun at 3000 rpm for 5 min. 200 µL of supernatant was transferred to a 96-shallow well micro titre plate, dried under nitrogen at 50 °C and reconstituted with 80 µL of 40% methanol in water. Plates were covered in foil and mixed gently for 10 min on a plate mixer before analysis.

2.6. LCMSMS Analysis

The LCMSMS system comprised an ultra high pressure liquid chromatography (UHPLC) quaternary pump combined with a TSQ Vantage mass spectrometer both from Thermo Fisher (Waltham, Mass., USA). An in-line Thermo Fisher turbulent flow (TLX) solid phase extraction was available for use. It comprised of a second UHPLC pump and a cyclone-P Turboflow™ (0.5 × 50 mm) extraction column. TLX technology works as follows. Prepared samples are injected onto the turboflow column at high flow rate using the first UHPLC pump (Loading pump). A combination of diffusion and size exclusion results in the retention of low molecular weight (<600 amu) polar and non-polar compounds. High molecular weight compounds are not retained and flow to waste. The turboflow column is then eluted with solvent and sample is transferred to an analytical column for chromatography separation and detection by mass spectrometry. The method removes protein particulates and phospholipids which can have a negative impact on analytical chromatography column performance and lifetime.

Solvent A consisted of ultra-pure water (Milliq, Merck, Darmstat, Germany) with 0.05% formic acid and 2 mM ammonium formate. Solvent B was 100% methanol. Solvent C was 100% acetonitrile. Solvent D was acetonitrile/isopropanol/acetone (45:45:10).

The turboflow UHPLC method contains a series of steps that control pump flow rate, valve positions, step duration and mobile phase composition. Briefly, the prepared samples were injected onto the turboflow column, via a 20 µL sample loop, at a flow rate of 1.5 mL/min (95% solvent A and 5% solvent C). Bound material was transferred to the analytical column by eluting the turboflow column with 80% acetonitrile from an inline elution loop at a low flow rate (0.1 mL/min) for 1 min. Chromatographic separation was achieved by ramping of mobile phase B to 90% in 5 min before holding for 1 min at 0.5 mL/min. During the chromatography phase the turboflow column was washed with 100% mobile phase D before the elution loop was refilled with 80% acetonitrile. The total run time was 9.15 min. Detailed chromatography settings are shown in Table A1.

The capillary voltage on the ion source was 3000 volts, the capillary temperature was 320 °C, the vaporiser temperature was 450 °C, sheath gas pressure was 50, ion sweep pressure 1.0 and auxiliary gas pressure 15 (arbitrary units). The quantifier precursor and product ions were 331.3 > 97.1 for 17 OHP and 339.3 > 100.1 for 17OHP-d_8. The qualifier ion transition for 17OHP was 331.3 > 109.1. The scan width was 0.050 m/z for each transition with a scan time of 0.020 s. The de-clustering voltage was 3 V.

2.7. LCMSMS Quantification

Data processing was performed using Tracefinder software provided with the instrument. Peak area ratios of 17OHP/17OHP-d_8 were plotted against standard concentrations to achieve a linear calibration curve plotted with a 1/X reciprocal fit weighting to ensure maximum accuracy at lower concentrations.

2.8. LCMSMS Assay Performance Assessment

Accuracy and recovery were assessed using reference material with known 17OHP enrichment supplied by the CDC. Recovery was calculated from the baseline 17OHP values, enriched values supplied with the samples and the LCMSMS results in 3 concentration levels. Within and between batch precision was assessed in 3 levels of control material prepared in the laboratory. Linearity was assessed using incremental quantities of calibration material. The influence of ion suppression was assessed by monitoring of a post column infusion of 17OHP-d_8 in 5 extracted bloodspots using a previously described procedure [11]. The lower limit of quantification (LOQ) was assessed by repeated analysis of enriched bloodspot samples with 17OHP concentrations of 1–10 nmol/L.

Newborn screening performance incorporating LCMSMS was determined by reviewing CAH newborn screening data (n = 117,063 neonates) 2 years after LCMSMS implementation. Data was compared to screening performance in newborns (n = 116,097) born in the 2 years prior to LCMSMS implementation.

2.9. Statistical Analysis and Comparison between LCMSMS and Immunoassay

The relationship between LCMSMS and immunoassay after solvent extraction was determined using methods described by Bland and Altman [12]. Difference plots were constructed using the mean percentage difference between LCMSMS and immunoassay for each specimen and the mean of both methods. The average difference and 2 standard deviation ranges for the limits of agreement were calculated.

The correlation between LCMSMS and immunoassay was determined in EQA proficiency material. Residual EQA specimens (n = 30) with concentration ranges spanning the primary screening cut-offs were subjected to LCMSMS. Solvent extraction was not carried out on these specimens because they were insufficient for second tier immunoassay measurement and they would not be expected to contain immunoassay interfering compounds.

The false positive rate, the sensitivity, specificity and positive predictive value of screening before and after LCMSMS implementation was determined. The Pearson's Chi squared test (X^2) was used to determine the significance of screening outcome and choice of second-tier method.

3. Results

3.1. LCMSMS Method Performance

Full chromatographic baseline separation for 17OHP from other potentially interfering isobaric compounds was achieved (Figure 1). Monitoring of the 17OHP internal standard response (m/z 339.25 > 100.2) in five extracted samples revealed no drop in internal standard response between 6.5 and 7.5 min (the elution time of 17OHP), an indication that ion suppression had little effect on 17OHP quantitation.

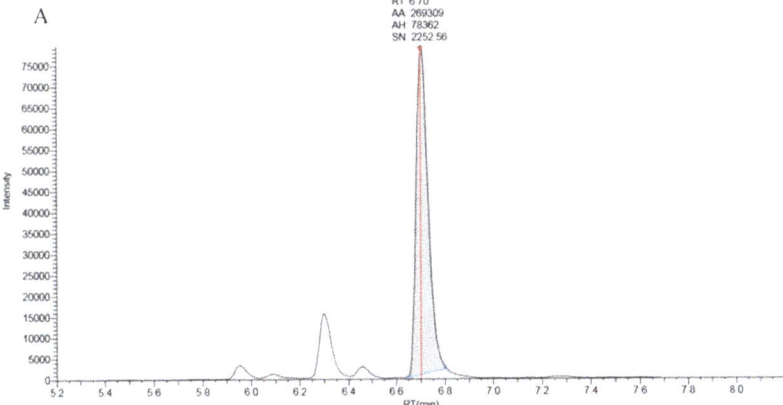

Figure 1. Cont.

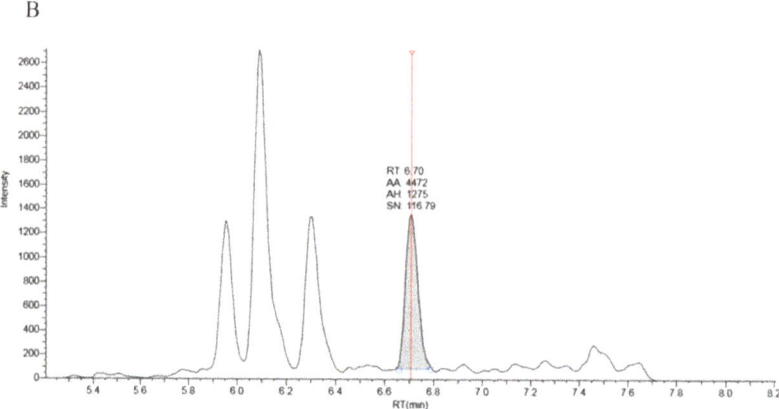

Figure 1. Chromatography traces for the 331.3 > 97.2 MRM signal by LCMSMS for **A**: True positive second tier LCMSMS screening test for CAH (17OHP = 401 nmol/L), **B**: Negative LCMSMS CAH screening test at day 2 on a baby born at 32 weeks gestation (17OHP = 7 nmol/L).

The average slope of 10 calibration curves carried out on separate days was 0.006711 (sd 0.000486) with a CV of 7.2%. Linearity was established up to 1600 nmol/L (r^2 = 0.999, Figure 2).

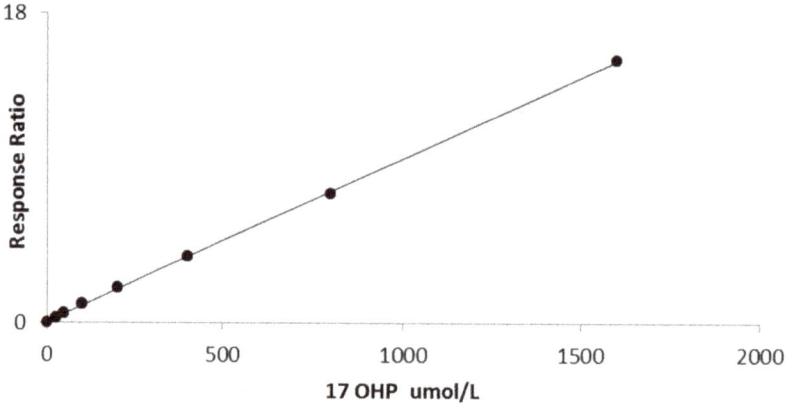

Figure 2. Linearity of bloodspot 17OHP by LCMSMS (r^2 = 0.999).

The average within batch precision was 9.1% (n = 20) with between batch precision of 9.1% (n = 22) across 3 levels of control material. Accuracy was within an average +2 nmol/L of 10 replicates of reference material with target ranges of 17 nmol/L, an average of −5 nmol/L with a target range of 82 nmol/L and an average of +2 nmol/L for a target range of 162 nmol/L (Table 1).

The average recovery for the method was 100.5% with a range of 98.6–102% at three bloodspot concentrations of 17OHP. The lower limit of quantification (LOQ) was defined as the lowest concentration of 17OHP with an inter-batch precision of <20%. The LOQ for 17OHP was determined to be 1 nmol/L. Results from analysis of 17-hydroxypregnenolone sulphate enriched bloodspots revealed no interference with 17OHP measurements (Table 2).

Table 1. Precision, Accuracy, bias and recovery data for 17OHP in bloodspots by LC-MSMS. * Target value assigned by the CDC. ** LCMSMS method mean ($n = 79$) from laboratories submitting analytical data to the CDC.

	Precision Data ($n = 24$)		
	Control 1	Control 2	Control 3
Within-Batch ($n = 20$)			
Mean (nmol/L)	14.6	74.9	155.7
CV%	13.7	7.0	6.2
Between-Batch ($n = 22$)			
Mean (nmol/L)	15.0	74.9	155.1
CV%	11.9	6.1	9.3
Accuracy			
	Level 1	Level 2	Level 3
CDC Target Value (nmol/L) *	15	66	134
Inter-laboratory Mean (nmol/L) **	17	82	162
Mean (nmol/L) ($n = 10$)	19	77	164
Recovery			
	Level 1	Level 2	Level 3
Baseline Level	ND	ND	ND
Enrichment (nmol/L)	15.2	76.0	152
Mean	15.0	74.9	155
Recovery (%)	101%	98.6%	102%

Table 2. Comparison of interferences from 17-hydroxpregnenolone sulphate.

17OH-Pregnenolone Sulphate Conc. (nmol/L)	Immunoassay17OHP (nmol/L)	LCMSMS17OHP (nmol/L)
500	2.8	<1
1000	5.8	<1
2000	8.8	<1
4000	23.5	<1

3.2. Correlation between LCMSMS and Immunoassay

Bland Altman analysis to determine the difference between LCMSMS and immunoassay in false positive neonatal screening samples revealed a mean difference of −36.1% with 2 standard deviation limits of agreement of −97.8% to 26.4% (Figure 3). Analysis in the true positive CAH screening samples revealed a mean difference of −45.5% with limits of agreement of −90.7% to 0.4%. Correlation of LCMSMS and immunoassay in EQA samples revealed a difference of −11.1% with limits of agreement between 38.8% and 27.6% (Figure 4). The Bland Altman plot regression line slopes for each sample group was not significantly different from 0 ($p > 0.05$), indicating an insignificant change in bias across the measured range for each group.

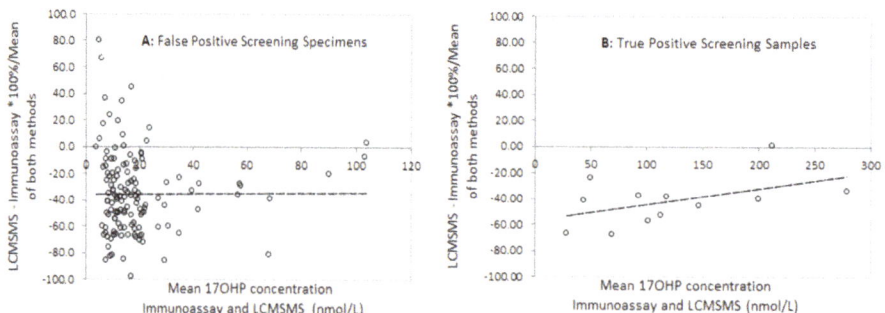

Figure 3. Bland Altman difference plots for LCMSMS and Immunoassay after solvent extraction for **A**: False positive screening Tests and **B**: True Positive Screening tests, and for LCMSMS and Immunoassay for External quality assurance samples. **A**: Slope = 0.02 ($p = 0.89$), mean difference = −35.7%, 2 sd limits of agreement (LOA) −97.9% to +26.4%); **B**: Slope = 0.13 ($p = 0.15$), mean difference = −45.5%, LOA= −90.7% to −0.4%).

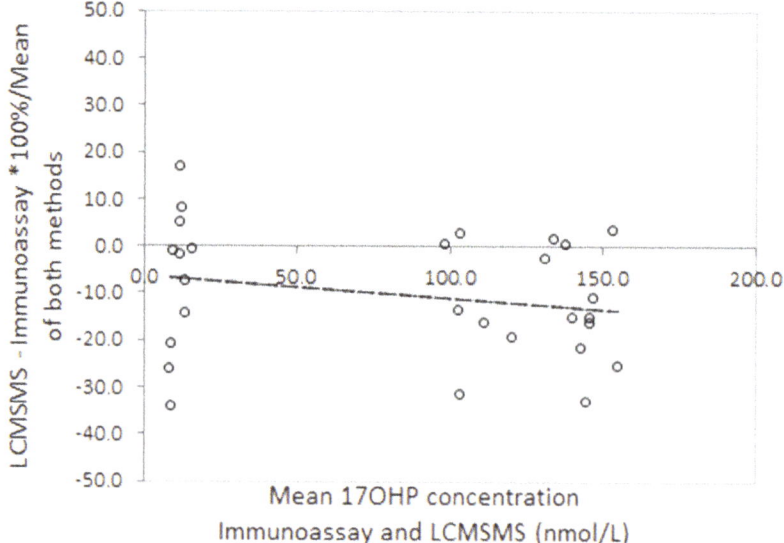

Figure 4. Bland Altman plots for LCMSMS and Immunoassay for external quality assurance samples ($n = 32$). Slope = −0.02 ($p = 0.52$), mean difference = −11.1%, LOA = −38.8 to 27.6%.

3.3. Analysis of Newborn Screening Data

During the 2 years prior to LCMSMS implementation 1643 s tier immunoassay tests were performed. Of these 362 samples were above the newborn screening cut-off with 175 positive screening results. During that time there were three clinically proven cases of P450c21 deficiency and 172 false positive tests requiring follow up. In the 2 years after LCMSMS implementation there were 1213 s tier LCMSMS tests with 113 samples above the screening cut-off resulting in 45 positive screens. Of these 5 were clinically confirmed cases of CAH due 21-hydroxylase deficiency and 40 were considered false positive tests requiring follow up. The data indicated there was a significant relationship between the second-tier method of analysis and the number of false positive screening results using the same newborn screening 17OHP cut-offs. (Pearsons Chi-Squared statistic, $X^2 = 47.29$, $p < 0.00001$, $n = 2856$). The positive predictive value of newborn screening for CAH due to 21-hydroxylase deficiency increased from 1.71% to 11.1% (Table 3) when LCMSMS was introduced. LCMSMS significantly improves screening specificity for CAH without any other changes to newborn screening protocols.

Table 3. Newborn Screening Metrics for CAH before and after LCMSMS Implementation.

	Immunoassay 2 nd Tier	LCMSMS 2 nd Tier
Start Date	1 December 2015	1 December 2017
End Date	30 November 2017	30 November 2019
Number of Babies Screened	117,063	116,097
Number of Specimens	118,624	117,624
Number of second tier tests	1643	1213
Number of 2 nd tier results above the screening cut-off	362	113
Number of positive screens	175	45
Number of true positive screens	3	5
Number of false positive screens	172	40
False Positive Rate	0.15%	0.03%
Specificity	99.85%	99.97%
Positive predictive Value	1.71%	11.11%

The birth weights, gestational age (GA) at birth, the age of sampling and 17OHP are shown in Table A2. The table also includes the corrected gestational age (GA at birth + age at sampling). The GA of babies at birth ranged from 23 to 36 weeks with corrected GA of 27–36 weeks. All false positive specimens were collected in hospital neonatal units or neonatal intensive care units. In total, 16 samples were from neonates screened under the low birth weight protocol. In total, 24 samples were from neonates screened under the single sample screening protocol. All neonates with a false positive screen were premature (<37 weeks gestational age).

4. Discussion

We have described a LCMSMS method to measure 17OHP in bloodspots as a second-tier test for newborn screening for CAH. The method was based on a procedure described by Rossi et al. [13] with an additional automated sample clean up step by turbulent flow solid phase extraction. Our inter assay method precision range of 9.3–11.9% was comparable to other reports (7.9–10.9% [10], 3.9–18% [14]). The method is also sufficiently accurate, particularly when using the inter laboratory method mean as a target for certified CDC material. The method was linear beyond the clinical requirements for CAH investigations. The mean recovery for three 17OHP concentrations was almost 100%, although a repeat recovery experiment in native blood to account for protein binding of 17OHP may be have been more appropriate. However, we assumed that protein precipitation would release bound 17OHP in the sample when the acetonitrile solution was added during the extraction phase of the procedure. There was no interference detected from sulphated steroids when added at concentrations expected in bloodspot specimens from very premature neonates. The limit of quantification was 1 nmol/L.

Salter et al. [9] and Janzen et al. [10] found poor correlation between LCMSMS and radioimmunoassay in a small number of CAH patient samples. When comparing the two techniques, Boelen et al. reported that LCMSMS measurements in neonatal samples were up to 75% lower than immunoassay [15], while Dhillon et al. showed that the difference between LCMSMS and immunoassay was much wider in very low birth weight babies [16]. Our data confirms their reports that LCMSMS 17OHP is significantly lower and the differences are highly variable, particularly in low birth weight babies.

The correlation between LCMSMS and immunoassay is improved when external quality assurance proficiency testing samples are used. LCMSMS is, on average, 11% lower than immunoassay. The reasons for this are unclear as the samples would not be expected to contain large quantities of cross reacting steroid precursor. There is evidence that sample disks taken from the outer edges of a bloodspot can have up to 25% lower concentrations of metabolites than sample disks taken from the centre of a bloodspot [17]. It is common practice in screening laboratories to punch disks from the centre of a bloodspot. During our method development the restricted quantities of residual EQA material and newborn screening specimens meant that disks where often taken from the outer edges of the bloodspot.

LCMSMS removes interference from other steroids but can be prone to interference from other isobaric steroids, a number of which can be present in newborn bloodspots. 11-deoxycorticosterone, an aldosterone precursor, has previously been shown to interfere with 17OHP measurements by LCMSMS [9] when present in large quantities. Although concentrations are normally much lower than 17OHP and even absent in 21-hydroxylase deficiency, we did not note any interfering peaks in our method in any of our specimens.

For newborn screening to be effective, positive tests need to be confirmed quickly so clinical referrals can be made. Our method allows LCMSMS to be carried out quickly after an initial elevated primary immunoassay test. Calibration stability suggests that periods between full method calibration only need to be performed every 10 days, therefore second-tier results will most often be available within 2 h when required.

This approach has significantly improved screening specificity for CAH in New Zealand. The number of false positive screening tests have fallen from 86 to 20 per year, a reduced burden on the screening programme and a reduction in screening interventions. False positive tests are expensive as they require follow up, sample recollection and analysis, and can cause lasting anxiety for families [18]. All of our false positive screening tests were from samples taken in specialist neonatal units in New Zealand hospitals. The risk of an undetected salt wasting crisis occurring in this group of babies is low, and a protocol that includes specimen collection at unit discharge, (i.e., at a corrected gestational age that is near-term) may reduce the false positive rate further.

The use of 17OHP and androstenedione expressed as a ratio to cortisol has been used as additional secondary marker in CAH [14,19,20]. In a report by Schwarz et al. on the use of LCMSMS incorporating 17OHP and a ratio of androstenedione plus 17OHP to cortisol (17OHP+A4/CORT) resulted in a significant reduction of the false positive rate in CAH screening from 2.64% to 0.09% over a 13 month period [20]. Using 17OHP alone, our data showed the false positive rate was reduced from 0.15% to 0.03% after the introduction of LCMSMS. The second tier 17OHP cut-off was higher in New Zealand (23–34 nmol/L) when compared to a 17OHP cut-off of 17.3 nmol/L (12.5 mg/mL serum equivalent). Additionally, the strategy for repeat sampling in low birth weight neonates in New Zealand may have contributed significantly to a lower false positive rate than a single sample approach at the same age (2–3 days). The protocols used by both programmes point to the broader issue of a lack of a common approach to CAH screening in general. Comparing screening performance is difficult when there is a lack of consensus across most CAH screening programmes for an approach to timing of sample collection, screening cut-offs, laboratory protocols, the definition of what constitutes a positive screening test and a definition of what form of CAH screening programmes are trying to detect in the newborn period.

There are however a number of additional analytical strategies that could be implemented to improve screening specificity further. The analysis of additional informative markers in CAH has been employed by measuring 17OHP with a combination of androstenedione, 11-deoxycortisol, 21-deoxycortisol, cortisol and several other steroids as a second tier test [10,13–16,19]. 21-deoxycortisol is emerging as a sensitive marker for CAH although it requires further evaluation [15]. Further evaluation of some of or all these markers to improve screening in New Zealand may be appropriate.

The National Newborn Metabolic Screening Programme in New Zealand is accredited under ISO15189 and is required to take part in external quality assessment. While a number of proficiency schemes for bloodspot 17OHP by immunoassay and LCMSMS are available worldwide, no regular scheme is available for bloodspots that include additional informative steroids outside of the United States. Our approach was to develop a LCMSMS method for 17OHP alone, evaluate its screening performance, while participating in regular external quality assessment using certified schemes. This has allowed the screening laboratory to gain technical experience of LCMSMS and to build a platform to add additional markers. Alternatively a small adjustment to the sampling protocols (e.g., a final sample collect at neonatal unit discharge) combined with a second tier LCMSMS 17OHP level may offer a more simple approach to optimising CAH screening specificity. Both of these strategies require further study.

Although LCMSMS analysis of 17OHP offers improved analytical specificity, the limited data from the true positive cases does not indicate a change in screening sensitivity. Screening in New Zealand targets the severe salt-wasting form of 21-hydroxylase deficiency, however neonates with the simple virilising form of the disorder are detected by the screening programme and benefit from early treatment. Some neonates with 21-hydroxylase deficiency in New Zealand have been missed by screening and presented later with the symptoms of androgen excess. Our method offers the potential to add additional markers to improve screening sensitivity. For example, 21-deoxycortisol has been shown to be a consistent marker for CAH in the neonatal period [15] and 11-deoxycortisol can be used to distinguish 21-hydroxylase deficiency from 11-hydroxylase deficiency which is present in approximately 5% of CAH cases [15]. A number of novel markers for CAH are emerging and there is considerable interest in role of 11-oxygenated 21-carbon steroids in CAH [21].

In summary, the replacement of immunoassay by LCMSMS as a second-tier test has significantly improved newborn screening specificity for CAH due to 21-hydroxylase deficiency in New Zealand. Small adjustments in a sampling protocols or additional steroid markers may contribute to improved specificity and sensitivity. Analysis of 17OHP in bloodspots is a simple and reliable procedure and results are available in the timeframes needed for clinical referral when required.

Author Contributions: Conceptualization, M.R.d.H., D.W., N.L.H., P.L.H.; methodology, M.R.d.H.; validation, M.R.d.H., T.P., L.G.B.; formal analysis, M.R.d.H.; investigation, M.R.d.H.; resources, M.R.d.H.; data curation, M.R.d.H., N.H.; writing—original draft preparation, M.R.d.H.; writing—review and editing, N.L.H., D.W., P.L.H.; visualization, M.R.d.H.; supervision, P.L.H., N.L.H., D.W. All authors have read and agreed to the published version of the manuscript.

Funding: This research received no external funding.

Conflicts of Interest: The authors declare no conflict of interest.

Appendix A

Table A1. Turboflow and Chromatography Conditions.

Step	Start	Seconds	Loading Pump (Turboflow)						Eluting Pump (Analytical)			
			Flow	Grad	%A	%B	%C	Tee	Loop	Flow	Grad	%A	%B
1	0.00	60	1.50	Step	95	5	-	-	out	0.50	Step	95	5
2	1.00	15	0.10	Step	95	5	-	-	out	0.40	Step	95	5
3	1.25	60	0.10	Step	95	5	-	T	in	0.40	Ramp	95	5
4	2.25	300	1.00	Step	-	-	100	-	in	0.50	Ramp	10	90
5	7.25	30	1.50	Step	20	80	-	-	in	0.50	Step	10	90
6	7.75	60	1.50	Step	95	5	-	-	out	0.50	Ramp	95	5
7	8.75	30	1.50	Step	95	5	-	-	out	0.50	Step	95	5

Table A2. Details of all Positive Newborn Screening Specimens Using LCMSMS as a Second Tier Test for Newborn Screening for CAH. *NNU = Neonatal Unit. **CGA = corrected gestational age, FP = false Positive, TP = True Positive.

No.	BW (g)	GA (wks)	CGA ** (wks)	Location *	Immun nmol/L	LCMSMS nmol/L	Screening Outcome
1	1900	32	32	NNU	74	23	FP
2	1765	33	33	NNU	60	23	FP
3	2180	33	33	NNU	43	23	FP
4	2482	33	34	NNU	45	23	FP
5	1950	34	35	NNU	110	23	FP

Table A2. Cont.

No.	BW (g)	GA (wks)	CGA ** (wks)	Location *	Immun nmol/L	LCMSMS nmol/L	Screening Outcome
6	2050	35	36	NNU	59	23	FP
7	2625	35	36	NNU	78	23	FP
8	2173	33	34	NNU	81	24	FP
9	1565	30	31	NNU	105	25	FP
10	1680	27	28	NNU	53	26	FP
11	1850	32	34	NNU	64	26	FP
12	2205	32	34	NNU	94	26	FP
13	2695	34	36	NNU	54	26	FP
14	1610	31	33	NNU	65	27	FP
15	2135	32	34	NNU	85	30	FP
16	2360	33	35	NNU	120	30	FP
17	1541	31	33	NNU	79	33	FP
18	1912	32	35	NNU	93	34	FP
19	1770	32	35	NNU	133	35	FP
20	1670	29	32	NNU	172	43	FP
21	1580	31	34	NNU	131	47	FP
22	2070	34	37	NNU	120	55	FP
23	2074	35	38	NNU	54	34	FP
24	2128	35	38	NNU	65	29	FP
25	1004	26	30	NNU	156	45	FP
26	870	28	32	NNU	56	36	FP
27	680	24	28	NNU	339	161	FP
28	835	25	29	NNU	130	36	FP
29	640	24	28	NNU	85	38	FP
30	610	24	28	NNU	136	70	FP
31	661	23	27	NNU	69	37	FP
32	655	26	31	NNU	108	44	FP
33	665	24	29	NNU	100	45	FP
34	653	24	29	NNU	102	47	FP
35	728	24	29	NNU	117	54	FP
36	614	24	29	NNU	178	96	FP
37	826	25	30	NNU	118	35	FP
38	733	27	32	NNU	73	36	FP
39	985	26	32	NNU	59	38	FP
40	680	24	30	NNU	149	50	FP
41	3975	38	38	Not stated	434	138	TP
42	3670	39	39	Not Stated	670	761	TP
43	2902	37	37	NNU	250	112	TP
44	3810	39	39	Not Stated	613	383	TP
45	3890	41	41	Not Stated	686	833	TP

References

1. Miller, W.L.; Auchus, R.J. The molecular biology, biochemistry, and physiology of human steroidogenesis and its disorders. *Endocr. Rev.* **2011**, *32*, 81–151. [CrossRef]
2. Hannon, W.H. *Clinical, Laboratory Standards I. Blood Collection on Filter Paper for Newborn Screening Programs: Approved Standard*; Clinical and Laboratory Standards Institute: Wayne, PA, USA, 2013.
3. Wong, T.; Shackleton, C.H.; Covey, T.R.; Ellis, G. Identification of the steroids in neonatal plasma that interfere with 17 alpha-hydroxyprogesterone radioimmunoassays. *Clin. Chem.* **1992**, *38*, 1830–1837.
4. Anandi, V.S.; Shaila, B. Evaluation of factors associated with elevated newborn 17-hydroxyprogesterone levels. *J. Pediatr. Endocrinol. Metab.* **2017**, *30*, 677–681. [CrossRef]
5. Ersch, J.; Beinder, E.; Stallmach, T.; Bucher, H.U.; Torresani, T. 17-Hydroxyprogesterone in premature infants as a marker of intrauterine stress. *J. Perinat. Med.* **2008**, *36*, 157–160. [CrossRef]
6. Fingerhut, R. False positive rate in newborn screening for congenital adrenal hyperplasia (CAH)-ether extraction reveals two distinct reasons for elevated 17 alpha-hydroxyprogesterone (17-OHP) values. *Steroids* **2009**, *74*, 662–665. [CrossRef]
7. Heather, N.L.; Seneviratne, S.N.; Webster, D.; Derraik, J.G.; Jefferies, C.; Carll, J.; Jiang, Y.; Cutfield, W.S.; Hofman, P.L. Newborn screening for congenital adrenal hyperplasia in New Zealand, 1994-2013. *J. Clin. Endocrinol. Metab.* **2015**, *100*, 1002–1008. [CrossRef]
8. Matern, D.; Tortorelli, S.; Oglesbee, D.; Gavrilov, D.; Rinaldo, P. Reduction of the false-positive rate in newborn screening by implementation of MS/MS-based second-tier tests: The Mayo Clinic experience (2004–2007). *J. Inherit. Metab. Dis.* **2007**, *30*, 585–592. [CrossRef]
9. Salter, S.J.; Cook, P.; Davies, J.H.; Armston, A.E. Analysis of 17 alpha-hydroxyprogesterone in bloodspots by liquid chromatography tandem mass spectrometry. *Ann. Clin. Biochem.* **2015**, *52*, 126–134. [CrossRef]
10. Janzen, N.; Peter, M.; Sander, S.; Steuerwald, U.; Terhardt, M.; Holtkamp, U.; Sander, J. Newborn screening for congenital adrenal hyperplasia: Additional steroid profile using liquid chromatography-tandem mass spectrometry. *J. Clin. Endocr. Metab.* **2007**, *92*, 2581–2589. [CrossRef]
11. Annesley, T.M. Ion suppression in mass spectrometry. *Clin. Chem.* **2003**, *49*, 1041–1044. [CrossRef]
12. Bland, J.M.; Altman, D.G. Statistical methods for assessing agreement between two methods of clinical measurement. *Lancet* **1986**, *1*, 307–310.
13. Rossi, C.; Calton, L.; Brown, H.A.; Gillingwater, S.; Wallace, A.M.; Petrucci, F.; Ciavardelli, D.; Urbani, A.; Sacchetta, P.; Morris, M. Confirmation of congenital adrenal hyperplasia by adrenal steroid profiling of filter paper dried blood samples using ultra-performance liquid chromatography-tandem mass spectrometry. *Clin. Chem. Lab. Med.* **2011**, *49*, 677–684.
14. Lacey, J.M.; Minutti, C.Z.; Magera, M.J.; Tauscher, A.L.; Casetta, B.; McCann, M.; Lymp, J.; Hahn, S.H.; Rinaldo, P.; Matern, D. Improved specificity of newborn screening for congenital adrenal hyperplasia by second-tier steroid profiling using tandem mass spectrometry. *Clin. Chem.* **2004**, *50*, 621–625. [CrossRef]
15. Boelen, A.; Ruiter, A.F.; Claahsen-van der Grinten, H.L.; Endert, E.; Ackermans, M.T. Determination of a steroid profile in heel prick blood using LC-MS/MS. *Bioanalysis* **2016**, *8*, 375–384. [CrossRef]
16. Dhillon, K.; Ho, T.; Rich, P.; Xu, D.D.; Lorey, F.; She, J.W.; Bhandal, A. An automated method on analysis of blood steroids using liquid chromatography tandem mass spectrometry: Application to population screening for congenital adrenal hyperplasia in newborns. *Clin. Chim. Acta* **2011**, *412*, 2076–2084. [CrossRef]
17. George, R.S.; Moat, S.J. Effect of Dried Blood Spot Quality on Newborn Screening Analyte Concentrations and Recommendations for Minimum Acceptance Criteria for Sample Analysis. *Clin. Chem.* **2016**, *62*, 466–475. [CrossRef]
18. Gurian, E.A.; Kinnamon, D.D.; Henry, J.J.; Waisbren, S.E. Expanded newborn screening for biochemical disorders: The effect of a false-positive result. *Pediatrics* **2006**, *117*, 1915–1921. [CrossRef]
19. Minutti, C.Z.; Lacey, J.M.; Magera, M.J.; Hahn, S.H.; McCann, M.; Schulze, A.; Cheillan, D.; Dorche, C.; Chace, D.H.; Lymp, J.F. Steroid profiling by tandem mass spectrometry improves the positive predictive value of newborn screening for congenital adrenal hyperplasia. *J. Clin. Endocr. Metab.* **2004**, *89*, 3687–3693. [CrossRef]

20. Schwarz, E.; Liu, A.; Randall, H.; Haslip, C.; Keune, F.; Murray, M.; Longo, N.; Pasquali, M. Use of Steroid Profiling by UPLC-MS/MS as a Second Tier Test in Newborn Screening for Congenital Adrenal Hyperplasia: The Utah Experience. *Pediatr. Res.* **2009**, *66*, 230–235. [CrossRef]
21. Turcu, A.F.; Nanba, A.T.; Chomic, R.; Upadhyay, S.K.; Giordano, T.J.; Shields, J.J.; Merke, D.P.; Rainey, W.E.; Auchus, R.J. Adrenal-derived 11-oxygenated 19-carbon steroids are the dominant androgens in classic 21-hydroxylase deficiency. *Eur. J. Endocrinol.* **2016**, *174*, 601–609. [CrossRef]

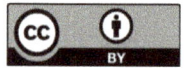

© 2020 by the authors. Licensee MDPI, Basel, Switzerland. This article is an open access article distributed under the terms and conditions of the Creative Commons Attribution (CC BY) license (http://creativecommons.org/licenses/by/4.0/).

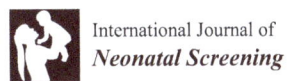

Article

Evaluation of a Two-Tier Screening Pathway for Congenital Adrenal Hyperplasia in the New South Wales Newborn Screening Programme

Fei Lai [1,2,*], Shubha Srinivasan [2,3] and Veronica Wiley [1,2]

1. Department of NSW Newborn Screening Programme, The Sydney Children Hospital Network, Westmead, NSW 2145, Australia; veronica.wiley@health.nsw.gov.au
2. Faculty of Medicine and Health, The University of Sydney Children's Hospital Westmead Clinical School, Westmead, NSW 2145, Australia; shubha.srinivasan@health.nsw.gov.au
3. Department of Endocrinology, The Sydney Children's Hospital Network, Westmead, NSW 2145, Australia
* Correspondence: fei.lai@health.nsw.gov.au

Received: 30 June 2020; Accepted: 7 August 2020; Published: 12 August 2020

Abstract: In Australia, all newborns born in New South Wales (NSW) and the Australia Capital Territory (ACT) have been offered screening for rare congenital conditions through the NSW Newborn Screening Programme since 1964. Following the development of the Australian Newborn Bloodspot Screening National Policy Framework, screening for congenital adrenal hyperplasia (CAH) was included in May 2018. As part of the assessment for addition of CAH, the national working group recommended a two-tier screening protocol determining 17α-hydroxyprogesterone (17OHP) concentration by immunoassay followed by steroid profile. A total of 202,960 newborns were screened from the 1 May 2018 to the 30 April 2020. A threshold level of 17OHP from first tier immunoassay over 22 nmol/L and/or top 2% of the daily assay was further tested using liquid chromatography tandem mass spectrometry (LC-MS/MS) steroid profiling for 17OHP (MS17OHP), androstenedione (A4) and cortisol. Samples with a ratio of (MS17OHP + A4)/cortisol > 2 and MS17OHP > 200 nmol/L were considered as presumptive positive. These newborns were referred for clinical review with a request for diagnostic testing and a confirmatory repeat dried blood spot (DBS). There were 10 newborns diagnosed with CAH, (9 newborns with salt wasting CAH). So far, no known false negatives have been notified, and the protocol has a sensitivity of 100%, specificity of 99.9% and a positive predictive value of 71.4%. All confirmed cases commenced treatment by day 11, with none reported as having an adrenal crisis by the start of treatment.

Keywords: congenital adrenal hyperplasia; newborn screening; 17-α hydroxyprogesterone; immunoassay; liquid chromatography tandem mass spectrometry; screening pathway

1. Introduction

Congenital adrenal hyperplasia (CAH) is an autosomal recessive disorder that occurs when there is a disruption in any of the enzymes along the adrenal steroidogenesis pathway [1–3]. CAH is categorised depending on which enzyme is affected. The severity of symptoms is inversely correlated with nonfunctioning enzyme activity [4]. The most common enzyme defect is 21-hydroxylase deficiency accounting for over 95% of cases. This form of CAH is subtyped into classical CAH and non-classical CAH. Classical CAH is further divided into salt-wasting CAH (SWCAH) and simple-virilising CAH (SVCAH) [4–6]. SWCAH, accounting for approximately 75% of classical CAH presentation, is the most severe form of CAH [7,8]. The incidence worldwide of classical CAH is usually considered to be approximately 1:14,000 to 1:18,000; however, it varies depending on the ethnic background [2]. Reported observed incidence is highest in Yupik Eskimos from Southern Alaska at 1:282 [9].

Newborn screening for CAH began with the development of a radioimmunoassay by Pang et al., 1977 [10] measuring 17 α-hydroxyprogesterone(17OHP) using blood on microfilter paper. Since then, worldwide CAH screening or pilot studies have ensued [11–22]. Newborn screening for CAH is aimed at identifying newborns with SWCAH promptly to prevent a life threatening adrenal crisis, thus reducing morbidity and mortality in affected individuals [23]. Detrimental adrenal and salt wasting crises occur within the first 2 to 3 weeks of life in newborns with SWCAH. Early clinical symptoms can be non-specific such as poor feeding, vomiting, diarrhoea and sepsis, which can lead to erroneous diagnoses [24]. Population newborn screening provides the opportunity to detect and treat those with CAH before the onset of significant symptoms.

Newborn bloodspot screening in Australia has been established since the late 1960s [25–27]. There are five state government-funded programs, which are located in Adelaide, Brisbane, Melbourne, Perth, and Sydney [28]. However, until recently New Zealand was the only center in Australasia screening for CAH [28]. In Australia, in New South Wales (NSW) and the Australia Capital Territory (ACT), a two-year pilot study was performed from 1st October 1995 to 30th September 1997, assessing the benefits and feasibility of screening CAH in newborns using an immunoassay for 17OHP with different follow-up action depending on birthweight and concentration of 17OHP compared to clinical diagnoses for newborns born in other states of Australia. Based on the findings from this study, implementing screening for CAH was considered justified [29]. However, funding for screening for CAH was not approved by the state governments. The decision was based on the concern of the harm caused by the number of false positive cases in the screened population as well as the evidence that the diagnosis for unsuspected cases in the screened population (median age: 13 days) was not significantly less than for the unscreened population (median age: 16 days).

In Australia, the inclusion of newborn screening for CAH was proposed to each state government at various times over the intervening years by the Australasian Pediatric Endocrine Group and the Human Genetic Society of Australasia (HGSA) [30]. A request was forwarded to the federal health minister in 2013. However, the process of adding CAH screening was challenging, as there was an absence of clear national policies or guidelines endorsed by all governments to support uniform newborn bloodspot screening. CAH was included as a recommended disorder in Australia in May 2018 due to the efforts of a time-limited multi-disciplinary CAH Assessment Working Group (CAHWG). The CAHWG also trialed the "Newborn Screening Bloodspot National Policy Framework", which included the tools for assessment of the inclusion or removal of recommended conditions [25].

The NSW Newborn Screening Programme commenced screening for CAH in May 2018 using the proposed recommended two-tier method protocol. This included all dried blood spot (DBS) samples being initially measured for 17-α hydroxyprogesterone (17OHP) using immunoassay followed by a second tier of steroid profiling using liquid chromatography tandem mass spectrometry (LC-MS/MS) for a percentage of samples with the highest 17OHP level. Whilst the CAHWG noted that the percentage could have differed in each state program, it was estimated to have been between 1 and 2% of sample results. This paper provides an evaluation of the first 2 years of implementation of screening for CAH in NSW.

2. Materials and Methods

2.1. Samples

All parents are provided with a multimedia information on newborn screening, including a pamphlet (Newborn Bloodspot Screening-Tests to Protect Your Baby) by the maternity health provider. Furthermore, educational videos and specific fact sheets are available on the website for parents and health professionals (https://www.schn.health.nsw.gov.au/find-a-service/laboratory-services/\protect\unhbox\voidb@x\hbox{newborn-screening}).

Newborn screening is not mandatory in Australia, and therefore following parent(s) consent, a heel prick blood spot sample is collected onto special pre-printed filter card provided by NSW

Newborn Screening Programme, ideally when the baby is 48 to 72 h after birth. The sample is air dried before being sent to the laboratory via a courier or local Australia Post. All DBS samples received in the laboratory by 10:15 am each day are processed as a batch on that working day.

Once received in the laboratory, the integrity and validity of each sample is determined. A repeat DBS sample is requested for samples that are deemed unsuitable due to being contaminated, insufficient or collected less than 24 h after birth, or having been collected after blood products were given to the newborn. A repeat sample is also requested at 1 month of age for any low birth weight (<1.5 kg) or premature (<30 weeks gestation) newborn. DBS samples with relevant clinical or family history information are processed for all routine screening tests plus assessed for further testing inclusion. Each initial DBS sample is allocated a unique laboratory sample identification number and with its corresponding demographic information entered into the laboratory information system (LabMaster Database) where a unique patient identification number is generated. Repeat samples received are matched with the previously generated unique patient identification number.

The DBS samples are then punched into 96 well microtiter plates using Panthera-Puncher™ 9 (Perkin Elmer, Turku, Finland) to simultaneously punch and distribute 3.2 mm blood disc into 6 different microtiter plates, one of which is a plate for immunoassay of 17αOHP.

2.2. Immunoassay

The concentration of 17OHP is initially determined on all DBS samples received using GSP® Neonatal 17 α-OH-Progesterone assay kit (PerkinElmer, Turku, Finland) on the 2021-0010 Genetic Screening Platform® (PerkinElmer, Turku, Finland) (GSP). The GSP assay is a competitive dissociation-enhanced lanthanide fluorescent immunoassay (DELFIA) (PerkinElmer, Turku, Finland). The kit provides the antibody-coated microtiter plates, calibrators, quality controls and all the reagents required to perform the immunoassay. A set of external quality control samples is also included in each daily assay. In our laboratory, the validation study for this kit using 5000 deidentified routine samples from full-term, normal birthweight infants established the 98th centile for 17OHP was 21.8 nmol/L whole blood. Therefore, samples with 17OHP ≥22 nmol/L and/or falling in the top 2% of all samples received for the daily assay for any birthweight were further tested using the second-tier LC-MS/MS steroid panel analysis. Samples with any clinical information or family history relevant to CAH were also tested using the LC-MS/MS steroid panel analysis.

2.3. LC-MS/MS

Unlabeled 17OHP, hydrocortisone and 4-Androstene-3,17-dione (A4) were obtained from LGC Dr. Ehrenstorfer GmbH (Augsburg, Germany). The isotopically labeled internal standard D8-17-OHP, [17-Hydroxyprogesterone(2,2,4,6,6,21,21,21-D8, 98%)], D7-Androstenedione, [4-Androstene-3,17-dione (2,2,4,6,6,16,16-D7, 97%)] and D4-Cortisol [Cortisol (9,11,12,123-D4, 98%)] (Cambridge Isotope Laboratories, Inc, Andover, MA, USA). Deep well microtiter plates (1000 µL) were supplied from LVL Technologies (Crailsheim, Germany), and microplate 96 plate pp flat bottom were supplied from Greiner Bio-One International (Frickenhausen, Germany). Fisher Chemical™ Optima™ LC-MS solvent from Thermo Fisher Scientific Australia Pty Ltd. (Victoria, Australia) and formic acid were obtained from Ajax Univar, Thermo Fisher Scientific (Victoria, Australia). Ammonium acetate suitable for mass spectrometry was supplied from Sigma Aldrich (WGK, Darmstadt, Germany).

The LC-MS/MS steroid assay for quantitation of 17OHP (MS17OHP), A4 and cortisol was a modified version of the assay from Rossi et al. [31]. The modifications were that stock for 17OHP, A4 and cortisol, and were made by dissolving unlabeled solid steroid compound in methanol:isopropanol (80:20 v/v) instead of ethanol; 75 µL of each calibrator was spotted onto filter cards rather than 25 µL; only one 3.2 mm blood disc was punched from each calibrator, control and sample and eluted with 220 µL of methanol:water (95:5 v/v) containing internal standards (deuterated 17OHP, A4 and cortisol) in a deep well polypropylene plate (1000 µL). The eluate was transferred to a 96 well flat bottom polypropylene plate and dried using warm air (40 °C) and reconstituted with 200 µL of methanol:water

(50:50 *v/v*) containing 2 nM ammonium acetate and 0.1% formic acid. Samples were analysed using ACQUITY XEVO®TQ-S (Waters, Milford, MA, USA). The ACQUITY XEVO TQS Targetlynx™ software (version 4.1, Waters, Milford, MA, USA) was used to calculate each steroid concentration. Results of steroid quantitation for a daily batch were available within 2 h. In our laboratory, the assay has proven to be robust and reproducible with a linear calibration curve ($r^2 = 0.99$) for all three steroid analytes and a coefficient variation of <10% for each of the three steroid analytes.

2.4. Criteria for and Follow-Up of an Abnormal Screen

A combination of the MS17OHP concentration and the ratio (17OHP + A4)/cortisol) was used to determine whether diagnostic testing was required. Newborns with a MS17OHP level >200 nmol/L or >25 nmol/L with a ratio of >2 were considered screen positive for CAH and referred for diagnostic testing. The pediatrician or general practitioner named on the DBS card was contacted to organize urgent further samples, including a repeat DBS sample and plasma, to quantitate electrolytes, glucose and a full steroid profile and to perform a clinical review of the baby. Figure 1 shows the analytical protocol. Results obtained by the screening laboratory were reviewed together with the diagnostic results and clinical evaluation to determine the diagnosis.

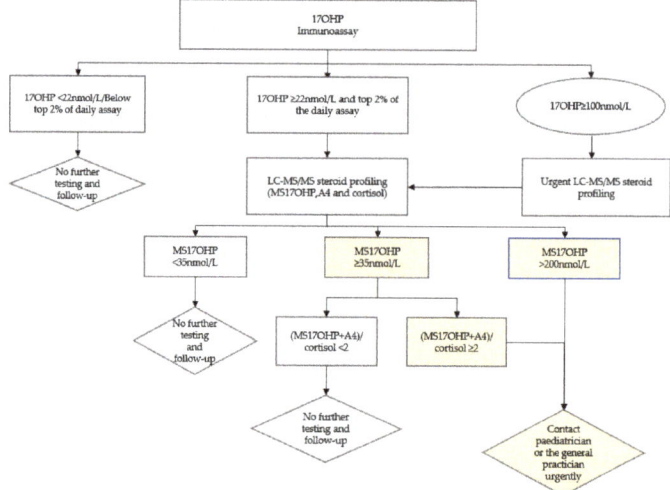

Figure 1. Analytical two-tier congenital adrenal hyperplasia (CAH) screening protocol using immunoassay as first tier followed by steroid profiling using liquid chromatography tandem mass spectrometry (LC-MS/MS) as a second-tier testing.

3. Results

There were 202,960 newborns tested during the period of May 2018 to April 2020, including 102,865 males. Of those screened, 2308 were from infants with very low birth weight (<1.5 kg). There were 206,469 samples, including the repeat dried blood spot collection (e.g., for screen positive, initial sample unsuitable or due to very low birthweight) analysed for 17OHP level using immunoassay. All samples were analysed for 17OHP level before day 8 of age with the exception of 0.02% of newborns with low birth weight and 0.22% of newborns with normal birth weight. Second-tier LC-MS/MS steroid profiling was required for 4218 samples after selecting the top 2% threshold of the daily immunoassay and any screen positive samples arising from the immunoassay. Of the total number from these samples, 927 (40.2%) newborns with very low birth weight and 2441 (1.2%) newborns with normal birthweight had a 17OHP level above 22 nmol/L.

Data collected showed that the 17OHP concentration from both immunoassay and LC-MS/MS obtained from newborns with very a low birth weight tended to be higher than that of the newborns with normal birth weight. Refer to Figure 2.

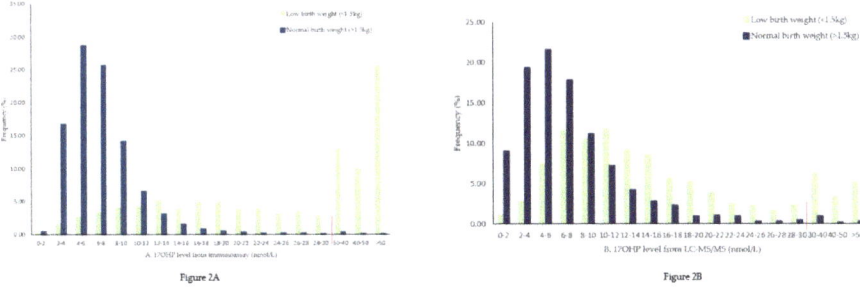

Figure 2A

Figure 2B

Figure 2. Distribution frequency of 17α-hydroxyprogesterone (17OHP) level. (**A**). 17OHP level (nmol/L) from immunoassay and (**B**). 17OHP level from LC-MS/MS.

The number of presumptive positive samples based solely on MS17OHP > 25 nmol/L was 241; however, after applying the ratio calculation of (MS17OHP + A4)/cortisol or for samples with MS17OHP > 200 nmol/L, there were 14 newborns who were deemed presumptive positive. Following diagnostic sample results and clinical review, 10 were proven to have CAH with 9 SWCAH and 1 newborn classified SVCAH. There was a higher proportion of males in the newborns (6/10) diagnosed with CAH.

Samples with clinical information supplied such as ambiguous genitalia, indeterminate sex and query CAH were also tested with LC-MS/MS steroid profiling regardless of the immunoassay 17OHP level. A total of 20 newborns had clinical information suggestive of CAH. Out of the 20 newborns, 17 newborns had an initial immunoassay result for 17OHP of less than 13 nmol/L and normal MS17OHP level. The other 3 newborns (case numbers 1, 5 and 7 in Tables 1 and 2) were confirmed to have CAH. All confirmed cases were initially notified by day 9 of life, and all had treatment commenced by day 20.

Table 1. Cases of CAH follow-up due to presumptive positive for New South Wales (NSW) Newborn Screening Programme from 1 May 2018 to 31 December 2019.

Case number	Sex	Birth Weight (kg)	Gestational Age (Days)	Initial DBS Sample Collection (*)	Initial DBS Sample Received Date (*)	Immuno-Assay 17OHP	Results from Steroid Profiling MS17OHP	A4	CORTISOL	Ratio	Initial Day of Notification (*)
1	I	3.51	287	2	5	>220	97	46	47	3	5
2	F	3.3	280	2	4	>220	>250	150	18	>22	4
3	F/tw2	1.66	238	2	7	>220	173	11	73	3	9
4	M	4.37	284	2	6	>220	228	148	23	16	6
5	F	2.91	266	2	6	>220	208	64	49	6	6
6	M	1.58	216	3	6	>220	403	30	31	14	6
7	M	3.97	266	2	4	>220	455	139	810	1	4
8	M	1.58	280	3	6	>220	403	30	31	14	6
9	F	0.68	175	2	5	100.3	104	51	63	2	5
10	M	4.5	287	3	8	>220	136	49	8	23	8
11	M	4.35	280	3	6	>220	364	297	26	25	6
12	F	2.55	238	2	6	90.7	46.1	7.1	22.7	2	6
13	M	2.03	252	2	7	45	34.8	4	10.5	4	7
14	M	0.49	175	3	6	180	55.2	13	24	3	6

Analytes are displayed in nmol/L whole blood; NFT-no further follow-up; (*) all samples collection and received date are calculated from date of birth, case number 3 is a female and twin number 2.

Table 2. Diagnostic results.

Case Number	Na *	K *	Glucose *	17OHP **	A4 **	CORTISOL **	TESTOSTERONE **	Family History	Symptoms	Diagnosis Suspected before Notification	Final Diagnosis	Treatment Commencement Day (*)
1	141	4.9		234		320	5.8	N	virilisation	Y	SW CAH	5
2	119	7.3	3.8	680	130	61		N	poor weight gain	N	SW CAH	11
3	130	6.1	30.3	212		86		N		N	SW CAH	9
4	136	5.8	4.2		>40		26.7	N		N	SW CAH	7
5	132	8	4.6	175	25	87	2.2	N	hypotension (associated with acute respiratory illness) virilisation	Y	SW CAH	7
6	133	5.7	3.8	>460	>37	104	51.4	N	poor feeding, preterm	N	SW CAH	8
7	136	5.3		652		88		Y	mild scrotal-transient, excess pigmentation	Y	SV CAH	2
8	133	5.7	3.8	>460	>37	104	51	N	poor feeding, preterm	N	SW CAH	8
9											NFT	
10	135	5.5	5	340	>38	31	3.5	N		N	SW CAH	10
11	132	7		498		64		N	lethargy	N	SW CAH	20
12	135	5.6	6.5	13		258					NFT	
13											NFT	
14											NFT	

* Analytes are displayed in mmol/L; ** analytes are displayed in nmol/L; case numbers 9, 13 and 14 only had a repeat dried blood spot recollection, and were clinically reviewed but had no plasma sample recollection; NFT-no further testing or follow-up; (*) days calculated from date of birth.

4. Discussion

Despite inclusion of screening for CAH in many newborn screening programs internationally, it has not been included in all developed programs. There remain reservations, as CAH can be detected through clinical assessment and there are noted to be high false-positive rates generated from immunoassay in low birth weight premature infants [22,32,33]. A study from the United Kingdom argued that screening for CAH has no impact on the morbidity and mortality of patients with CAH and therefore does not include CAH in its screening program [34]. It has also been suggested that newborn screening for CAH only benefits male newborns, as females can be clinically detected due to virilisation [35]. However, countries around the world screening for CAH have demonstrated that the benefits from early detection of newborns with CAH include reducing morbidity and mortality, especially for newborns with SWCAH, and can assist in gender assignment for newborn with SVCAH [36].

There have been several strategies implemented by screening programs to improve the specificity of CAH screening. Improvement in the specificity was observed when the cut-off level of 17OHP was stratified based on either gestational age or birth weight and/or age of sampling [1,14,16,18,37–40]. Although gestational age stratification of 17OHP concentration was shown to give higher specificity, birth weight stratification has been more widely used [22,41,42]. However, even with the implementation of these strategies, 1% of newborn may require recollection [40]. Similarly, in NSW a two-year pilot program from 1st October 1995 to 30th September 1997 [29] showed that despite stratified action limits for low birth weight newborns there were 6% of infants <2 kg birth weight requiring further sample collection compared to 0.3% of infants with birth weight >2 kg. In an effort to simplify the potential use of multiple action limits and assess the expected total workload for each state program, the CAHWG recommended the use of a percentile cut-off for referral to second tier without stratification due to birth weight or gestational age [43]. By performing a second-tier assay on the top 2% of the daily samples received, our laboratory screening of ~100,000 newborns per year was an average required to test 8 samples by steroid profile each day, which could have been reduced to 5 to 6 depending on the stratified action limits. The time difference and cost for processing 8 versus 5 samples was deemed insignificant.

The use of a second-tier LC-MS/MS steroid profile was first presented by Lacey et al. measuring 17OHP, A4 and cortisol [24]. By incorporating a second tier of steroid profiling using LC-MS/MS and the use of (MS17OHP + A4)/cortisol) ratio, the NSW Newborn Screening Programme has successfully screened over 200,000 newborns for CAH. In order to simplify the test cascade algorithm, it was determined that 2% of the daily population of samples would be tested with the second-tier assay. During initial evaluation of the 17OHP immunoassay on 5000 samples, the 98th centile of those with a birth weight >1.5 kg was 22 nmol/L whole blood. Therefore, to ensure all samples received that would be in the top 2% of a year, all samples with 17OHP >22 nmol/L were further tested. Using this protocol 14 newborns required further samples. There were 10 newborns diagnosed with CAH after diagnostic testing and a full clinical review: 1 SVCAH; 9 SWCAH (5 males, 3 females and 1 indetermine sex (chromosomally female)). All 9 infants with SWCAH had no prior family history of CAH, although 3 (cases 1, 5 and 7) of the newborns did have clinical observations noted on the DBS sample (Tables 1 and 2). The newborn with SVCAH (case 7) had a family history of CAH. Although this newborn had a steroid ratio of 1, the MS17OHP level was grossly elevated, prompting further follow-up action.

The four presumptive positive newborns requiring additional follow-up due to abnormal ratio were all deemed to be normal after either a DBS sample recollection, clinical review or diagnostic testing, and all remain well. Two of the newborns were extremely premature (Table 1). The protocol used therefore only provided a few false positives (4/202,960) and had no known false-negative results. We also successfully notified likely CAH cases before any of the newborns presented with an adrenal crisis.

There have been various studies investigating the feasibility of increasing the number of analytes in the steroid panel to increase specificity and sensitivity [44–48]. There are studies that show that the inclusion of 21-deoxycortisol and 11-deoxycortisol is more specific for detecting SWCAH by excluding β-hydroxylase deficiency [47–50]. Investigation of additional ratios (i.e., 17OHP + 21-deoxycortisol/cortisol) has been shown to be specific for 21 hydroxylase deficiency [49]. Further studies will be carried out to determine if the addition of 21-deoxycortisol and 11-deoxycortisol will be beneficial to our screening program.

SWCAH can present with a life-threatening adrenal crisis within the first two weeks of life [51]. Screening for CAH, notification of suspicion and diagnosis needs to be achieved before a potential adrenal crisis occurs. Using the two-tiered protocol, all suspected cases of CAH were notified by day 9 of life.

The gene that encodes the 21-hydroxylase enzyme is CYP21A2. Molecular analysis of CYP21A2 variant is hampered by the difficulty of isolating the highly homologous pseudogene CYP21A1P from the active CYP21A2 gene. Further, current molecular assays require at least 2 days to provide results, therefore the length of time to generate results is a deterrent for newborn screening [36,52]. However, variant analysis of the CYP21A2 gene has the potential for further increasing the specificity and sensitivity for screening CAH by basing it on genotype/phenotype studies. Biochemical analysis interferences, such as prematurity or stress of newborns and assay steroid cross reactivity, do not affect molecular variant analysis [53]. Variant analysis has been reported to be able to further discriminate SVCAH from SWCAH [53]; however, so far the literature suggests that variant analysis has only been used as an adjunct for screening [36]. This may change in the near future as technologies advance, for example, using next-generation sequencing for the CYP21A2 gene was reported to be cost effective and less time consuming [54]. Therefore, the emergence of targeted next-generation sequencing should be explored as a feasible screening option.

In conclusion, by following the recommended screening pathway from the national newborn bloodspot policy, the NSW Newborn Screening Programme has successfully screened over 200,000 newborns for CAH detecting an incidence of SWCAH of 1:22,551. We achieved a 100% sensitivity and a specificity of 99.9%, and the positive predictive value was 71.4%. All newborns screened with positive SWCAH were notified before any adrenal crisis occurred, thereby reducing the need for intensive care intervention.

Author Contributions: Conceptualization, V.W.; methodology, V.W.; writing—original draft preparation, F.L.; writing—review and editing, V.W. and S.S.; All authors have read and agreed to the published version of the manuscript.

Funding: This research received no external funding.

Acknowledgments: The author would like to acknowledge everyone in the department of NSW Newborn Screening Programme for their contributions.

Conflicts of Interest: The authors declare no conflict of interest.

References

1. Speiser, P.W.; Arlt, W.; Auchus, R.J.; Baskin, L.S.; Conway, G.S.; Merke, D.P.; Meyer-Bahlburg, H.F.L.; Miller, W.L.; Murad, M.H.; Oberfield, S.E.; et al. Congenital adrenal hyperplasia due to steroid 21-hydroxylase deficiency: An endocrine society clinical practice guideline. *J. Clin. Endocrinol. Metab.* **2018**, *103*, 4043–4088. [CrossRef] [PubMed]
2. Witchel, S.F.; Azziz, R. Congenital adrenal hyperplasia. *J. Pediatric Adolesc. Gynecol.* **2011**, *24*, 116–126. [CrossRef] [PubMed]
3. Hannah-Shmouni, F.; Chen, W.; Merke, D.P. Genetics of congenital adrenal hyperplasia. *Endocrinol. Metab. Clin. N. Am.* **2017**, *46*, 435–458. [CrossRef] [PubMed]
4. Simpson, H.; Hughes, I. Congenital adrenal hyperplasia. *Medicine* **2017**, *45*, 502–505. [CrossRef]
5. Speiser, P.W.; White, P.C. Congenital adrenal hyperplasia. *N. Engl. J. Med.* **2003**, *349*, 776–788. [CrossRef]

6. Wass, J.A.H.; Stewart, P.M. *Oxford Textbook of Endocrinology and Diabetes*; Oxford University Press: Oxford, UK, 2011.
7. Nimkarn, S.G.P.; Yau, M.; New, M.I. *21-Hydroxylase Deficiency Congenital Adrenal Hyperplasia*; University of Washington: Seattle, WA, USA, 2016.
8. Nimkarn, S.; Lin-Su, K.; New, M.I. Steroid 21 hydroxylase deficiency congenital adrenal hyperplasia. *Pediatr. Clin. N. Am.* **2011**, *58*, 1281–1300. [CrossRef]
9. Pang, S.Y. Worldwide experience in newborn screening for classical congenital adrenal hyperplasia due to 21-hydroxylase deficiency. *Pediatrics* **1988**, *81*, 866. [CrossRef]
10. Pang, S.; Hotchkiss, J.; Drash, A.L.; Levine, L.S.; New, M.I. Microfilter paper method for 17α-hydroxyprogesterone radioimmunoassay: Its application for rapid screening for congenital adrenal hyperplasia. *J. Clin. Endocrinol. Metab.* **1977**, *45*, 1003–1008. [CrossRef]
11. Gong, L.-F.; Gao, X.; Yang, N.; Zhao, J.-Q.; Yang, H.-H.; Kong, Y.-Y. A pilot study on newborn screening for congenital adrenal hyperplasia in Beijing. *J. Pediatr. Endocrinol. Metab.* **2019**, *32*, 253–258. [CrossRef]
12. Heather, N.L.; Seneviratne, S.N.; Webster, D.; Derraik, J.G.B.; Jefferies, C.; Carll, J.; Jiang, Y.; Cutfield, W.S.; Hofman, P.L. Newborn screening for congenital adrenal hyperplasia in New Zealand, 1994–2013. *J. Clin. Endocrinol. Metab.* **2015**, *100*, 1002–1008. [CrossRef]
13. Kumar, R.K.; Das, H.; Kini, P. Newborn screening for congenital adrenal hyperplasia in India: What do we need to watch out for? *J. Obstet. Gynecol. India* **2016**, *66*, 415–419. [CrossRef] [PubMed]
14. Kopacek, C.; de Castro, S.M.; Prado, M.J.; da Silva, C.M.D.; Beltrão, L.A.; Spritzer, P.M. Neonatal screening for congenital adrenal hyperplasia in Southern Brazil: A population based study with 108,409 infants. *BMC Pediatr.* **2017**, *17*, 22. [CrossRef] [PubMed]
15. Pang, S.; Murphey, W.; Levine, L.S.; Spence, D.A.; Leon, A.; LaFranchi, S.; Surve, A.S.; New, M.I. A pilot newborn screening for congenital adrenal hyperplasia in Alaska. *J. Clin. Endocrinol. Metab.* **1982**, *55*, 413–420. [CrossRef] [PubMed]
16. Pearce, M.; DeMartino, L.; McMahon, R.; Hamel, R.; Maloney, B.; Stansfield, D.-M.; McGrath, E.C.; Occhionero, A.; Gearhart, A.; Caggana, M.; et al. Newborn screening for congenital adrenal hyperplasia in New York State. *Mol. Genet. Metab. Rep.* **2016**, *7*, 1–7. [CrossRef]
17. Perrin, C.W. Neonatal screening for congenital adrenal hyperplasia. *Nat. Rev. Endocrinol.* **2009**, *5*, 490.
18. Sarafoglou, K.; Gaviglio, A.; Hietala, A.; Frogner, G.; Banks, K.; McCann, M.; Thomas, W. Comparison of newborn screening protocols for congenital adrenal hyperplasia in preterm infants. *J. Pediatr.* **2014**, *164*, 1136–1140. [CrossRef]
19. Therrell, B.L.; Adams, J. Newborn screening in North America. *J. Inherit. Metab. Dis.* **2007**, *30*, 447–465. [CrossRef]
20. Tsuji-Hosokawa, A.; Konishi, K.; Hasegawa, S.; Anazawa, A.; Onishi, T.; Ono, M.; Morio, T.; Kitagawa, T.; Kashimada, K. Newborn screening for congenital adrenal hyperplasia in Tokyo, Japan from 1989 to 2013: A retrospective population-based study. *BMC Pediatr.* **2015**, *15*, 1–8. [CrossRef]
21. Van Der Kamp, H.J.; Noordam, C.; Elvers, B.; Van Baarle, M.; Otten, B.J.; Verkerk, P.H. Newborn screening for congenital adrenal hyperplasia in The Netherlands. *Pediatrics* **2001**, *108*, 1320–1324. [CrossRef]
22. Van der Linde, A.A.A.; Schönbeck, Y.; van der Kamp, H.J.; Akker, E.L.V.D.; van Albada, M.E.; Boelen, A.; Finken, M.J.J.; Hannema, S.E.; Hoorweg-Nijman, G.; Odink, R.J.; et al. Evaluation of the Dutch neonatal screening for congenital adrenal hyperplasia. *Arch. Dis. Child.* **2019**, *104*, 653–657. [CrossRef]
23. Pang, S.; Clark, A.; Neto, E.C.; Giugliani, R.; Dean, H.; Winter, J.; Dhondt, J.-L.; Farriaux, J.; Graters, A.; Cacciari, E.; et al. Congenital adrenal hyperplasia due to 21-hydroxylase deficiency: Newborn screening and its relationship to the diagnosis and treatment of the disorder. *Screening* **1993**, *2*, 105–139. [CrossRef]
24. Lacey, J.M.; Minutti, C.Z.; Magera, M.J.; Tauscher, A.L.; Casetta, B.; McCann, M.; Lymp, J.; Hahn, S.H.; Rinaldo, P.; Matern, D. Improved specificity of newborn screening for congenital adrenal hyperplasia by second-tier steroid profiling using tandem mass spectrometry. *Clin. Chem.* **2004**, *50*, 621–625. [CrossRef] [PubMed]
25. 12118_Newborn Bloodspot Framework_V4_WEB.PDF. Available online: http://www.cancerscreening.gov.au/internet/screening/publishing.nsf/Content/C79A7D94CB73C56CCA257CEEE0000EF35/$File/12118_Newborn%20Bloodspot%20Framework_V4_WEB.PDF (accessed on 29 June 2020).
26. Wudy, S.; Schuler, G.; Guijo, A.S.; Hartmann, M. The art of measuring steroids: Principles and practice of current hormonal steroid analysis. *J. Steroid Biochem. Mol. Boil.* **2018**, *179*, 88–103. [CrossRef] [PubMed]

27. Wilcken, B.; Wiley, V. Fifty years of newborn screening. *J. Paediatr. Child Heal.* **2015**, *51*, 103–107. [CrossRef]
28. Wilcken, B.; Wiley, V. Newborn screening. *Pathology* **2008**, *40*, 104–115. [CrossRef]
29. Gleeson, H.K.; Wiley, V.; Wilcken, B.; Elliott, E.J.; Cowell, C.; Thonsett, M.; Byrne, G.; Ambler, G. Two-year pilot study of newborn screening for congenital adrenal hyperplasia in New South Wales compared with nationwide case surveillance in Australia. *J. Paediatr. Child Heal.* **2008**, *44*, 554–559. [CrossRef] [PubMed]
30. Warne, G.L.; Armstrong, K.L.; Faunce, T.; Wilcken, B.M.; Boneh, A.; Geelhoed, E.; Craig, M.E. The case for newborn screening for congenital adrenal hyperplasia in Australia. *Med. J. Aust.* **2010**, *192*, 107. [CrossRef]
31. Rossi, C.; Calton, L.; Brown, H.A.; Gillingwater, S.; Wallace, A.M.; Petrucci, F.; Ciavardelli, D.; Urbani, A.; Sacchetta, P.; Morris, M.R. Confirmation of congenital adrenal hyperplasia by adrenal steroid profiling of filter paper dried blood samples using ultra-performance liquid chromatography-tandem mass spectrometry. *Clin. Chem. Lab. Med.* **2011**, *49*, 677–684. [CrossRef]
32. White, P.C. Optimizing newborn screening for congenital adrenal hyperplasia. *J. Pediatr.* **2013**, *163*, 10–12. [CrossRef]
33. Turcu, A.F.; Auchus, R.J. The next 150 years of congenital adrenal hyperplasia. *J. Steroid Biochem. Mol. Boil.* **2015**, *153*, 63–71. [CrossRef]
34. Hird, B.E.; Tetlow, L.; Tobi, S.; Patel, L.; Clayton, R. No evidence of an increase in early infant mortality from congenital adrenal hyperplasia in the absence of screening. *Arch. Dis. Child.* **2014**, *99*, 158–164. [CrossRef] [PubMed]
35. Van Vliet, G.; Czernichow, P. Screening for neonatal endocrinopathies: Rationale, methods and results. *Semin. Neonatol.* **2004**, *9*, 75–85. [CrossRef]
36. Speiser, P.W.; Azziz, R.; Baskin, L.S.; Ghizzoni, L.; Hensle, T.W.; Merke, D.P.; Meyer-Bahlburg, H.F.L.; Miller, W.L.; Montori, V.M.; Oberfield, S.E.; et al. Congenital adrenal hyperplasia due to steroid 21-hydroxylase deficiency: An Endocrine Society clinical practice guideline. *J. Clin. Endocrinol. Metab.* **2010**, *95*, 4133–4160. [CrossRef] [PubMed]
37. Hayashi, G.Y.; Carvalho, D.F.; De Miranda, M.C.; Faure, C.; Vallejos, C.; Brito, V.N.; Rodrigues, A.D.S.; Madureira, G.; Mendonca, B.B.; Bachega, T.A. Neonatal 17-hydroxyprogesterone levels adjusted according to age at sample collection and birthweight improve the efficacy of congenital adrenal hyperplasia newborn screening. *Clin. Endocrinol.* **2017**, *86*, 480–487. [CrossRef]
38. Chan, C.L.; McFann, K.; Taylor, L.; Wright, D.; Zeitler, P.; Barker, J. Congenital adrenal hyperplasia and the second newborn screen. *J. Pediatr.* **2013**, *163*, 109–113. [CrossRef]
39. Votava, F.; Novotna, D.; Kracmar, P.; Vinohradska, H.; Stahlova-Hrabincova, E.; Vrzalová, Z.; Neumann, D.; Malikova, J.; Lebl, J.; Matern, D. Lessons learned from 5 years of newborn screening for congenital adrenal hyperplasia in the Czech Republic: 17-hydroxyprogesterone, genotypes, and screening performance. *Eur. J. Nucl. Med. Mol. Imaging* **2012**, *171*, 935–940. [CrossRef]
40. Dörr, H.G.; Odenwald, B.; Nennstiel-Ratzel, U. Early diagnosis of children with classic congenital adrenal hyperplasia due to 21-hydroxylase deficiency by newborn screening. *Int. J. Neonatal Screen.* **2015**, *1*, 36–44. [CrossRef]
41. Gidlöf, S.; Wedell, A.; Guthenberg, C.; von Döbeln, U.; Nordenström, A. nationwide neonatal screening for congenital adrenal hyperplasia in Sweden. *JAMA Pediatr.* **2014**, *168*, 567. [CrossRef]
42. Van der Kamp, H.J.; Oudshoorn, C.G.M.; Elvers, B.H.; Van Baarle, M.; Otten, B.J.; Wit, J.; Verkerk, P.H. Cutoff levels of 17-α-hydroxyprogesterone in neonatal screening for congenital adrenal hyperplasia should be based on gestational age rather than on birth weight. *J. Clin. Endocrinol. Metab.* **2005**, *90*, 3904–3907. [CrossRef]
43. Congenital adrenal hyperplasia (CAH) condition assessment summary—March 2019.pdf. Available online: https://www.google.com.hk/url?sa=t&rct=j&q=&esrc=s&source=web&cd=&ved=2ahUKEwiH7MSEzpTrAhUqyosBHbNVBCQQFjAAegQIAhAB&url=http%3A%2F%2Fwww.cancerscreening.gov.au%2Finternet%2Fscreening%2Fpublishing.nsf%2FContent%2FC79A7D94CB73C56CCA257CEE0000EF35%2F%24File%2FCongenital%2520adrenal%2520hyperplasia%2520(CAH)%2520condition%2520assessment%2520summary%2520-%2520March%25202019.pdf&usg=AOvVaw0lv0qPSTCr6j5LW7p2zRCQ (accessed on 29 June 2020).
44. Guran, T.; Tezel, B.; Gürbüz, F.; Eklioğlu, B.S.; Hatipoğlu, N.; Kara, C.; Şimşek, E.; Çizmecioğlu, F.M.; Ozon, A.; Baş, F.; et al. Neonatal screening for congenital adrenal hyperplasia in Turkey: A pilot study with 38,935 infants. *J. Clin. Res. Pediatr. Endocrinol.* **2019**, *11*, 13–23. [CrossRef]

45. Choi, R.; Park, H.-D.; Oh, H.J.; Lee, K.; Song, J.; Lee, S. Dried blood spot multiplexed steroid profiling using liquid chromatography tandem mass spectrometry in Korean neonates. *Ann. Lab. Med.* **2019**, *39*, 263–270. [CrossRef] [PubMed]
46. Bialk, E.R.; Lasarev, M.R.; Held, P.K. Wisconsin's screening algorithm for the identification of newborns with congenital adrenal hyperplasia. *Int. J. Neonatal Screen.* **2019**, *5*, 33. [CrossRef]
47. Tieh, P.Y.; Yee, J.K.; Hicks, R.; Mao, C.S.-M.; Lee, W.-N. Utility of a precursor-to-product ratio in the evaluation of presumptive positives in newborn screening of congenital adrenal hyperplasia. *J. Perinatol.* **2017**, *37*, 283–287. [CrossRef] [PubMed]
48. Boelen, A.; Ruiter, A.F. Determination of a steroid profile in heel prick blood using LC-MSMS. *Bioanalysis* **2016**, *8*, 375–384. [CrossRef]
49. Janzen, N.; Peter, M.; Steuerwald, U.; Terhardt, M.; Holtkamp, U.; Sander, S. Newborn screening for congenital adrenal hyperplasia: Additional steroid profile using liquid chromatography-tandem mass spectrometry. *J. Clin. Endocrinol. Metab.* **2007**, *92*, 2581–2589. [CrossRef]
50. Hicks, R.A.; Yee, J.K.; Mao, C.S.; Graham, S.; Kharrazi, M.; Lorey, F.; Lee, W.P. Precursor-to-product ratios reflect biochemical phenotype in congenital adrenal hyperplasia. *Metabolomics* **2014**, *10*, 123–131. [CrossRef]
51. El-Maouche, D.; Arlt, W.; Merke, D.P. Congenital adrenal hyperplasia. *Lancet* **2017**, *390*, 2194–2210. [CrossRef]
52. Pignatelli, D.; Carvalho, B.L.; Palmeiro, A.; Barros, A.; Guerreiro, S.G.; Maçut, D. The complexities in genotyping of congenital adrenal hyperplasia: 21-hydroxylase deficiency. *Front. Endocrinol.* **2019**, *10*, 10. [CrossRef]
53. Sarafoglou, K.; Lorentz, C.P.; Otten, N.; Oetting, W.S.; Grebe, S.K.G. Molecular testing in congenital adrenal hyperplasia due to 21?-hydroxylase deficiency in the era of newborn screening. *Clin. Genet.* **2012**, *82*, 64–70. [CrossRef]
54. Turan, I.; Tastan, M.; Boga, D.D.; Gurbuz, F.; Kotan, L.D.; Tuli, A.; Yuksel, B. 21-Hydroxylase deficiency: Mutational spectrum and genotype–phenotype relations analyses by next-generation sequencing and multiplex ligation-dependent probe amplification. *Eur. J. Med. Genet.* **2019**, *63*, 103782. [CrossRef]

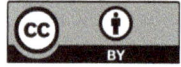

© 2020 by the authors. Licensee MDPI, Basel, Switzerland. This article is an open access article distributed under the terms and conditions of the Creative Commons Attribution (CC BY) license (http://creativecommons.org/licenses/by/4.0/).

MDPI
St. Alban-Anlage 66
4052 Basel
Switzerland
Tel. +41 61 683 77 34
Fax +41 61 302 89 18
www.mdpi.com

Actuators Editorial Office
E-mail: actuators@mdpi.com
www.mdpi.com/journal/IJNS

www.ingramcontent.com/pod-product-compliance
Lightning Source LLC
LaVergne TN
LVHW070606100526
838202LV00012B/576